BLACK WOMAN HEAL THY SELF

BLACK WOMAN HEAL THY SELF

*Obtain Your Ideal Level
of Wellbeing Your Way*

JENDAYI A. STAFFORD, PH.D.

*Carolyn Hubert-Black, Natalie Martin,
Anita Monique*

Contents

i

Disclaimer

This publication contains the opinions and ideas of its author(s). It is intended to provide helpful and informative material on the subjects addressed in the publication. It is sold with the understanding that the author(s) and publisher are not engaged in rendering medical, health, or any other kind of personal professional services in the book. The reader should consult his or her medical, health, or other competent professional before adopting any of the suggestions in this book or drawing inferences from it. This book also is not intended to serve as the basis for any financial decision, as a recommendation of a specific investment, or as an offer to sell or purchase any security.

Throughout this book, the author(s) may discuss several companies and entities in which the author(s) have a financial interest, and such interests are disclosed when those entities are first mentioned.

The author(s) and publisher specifically disclaim all responsibility for any liability, loss, or risk, personal or otherwise, which is incurred as a consequence, directly or indirectly, of the use and application of any of the contents of this book.

ii

Note to Readers

Every effort was made to ensure the accuracy of the information contained in this book as of the date of its publication. Please note that this book is not a comprehensive guide to all naturopathic medicines that exist for all conditions. Only select information was included in this book.

Due to the rate at which conditions change and new information and research are being published, the author(s) reserve the right to alter and update their opinions at any time. Although there is information in this book that is based on evidence-based practices and scientific research, other information provided in this book is based on the over 50 combined years of experience in studying naturopathic medicines and personal successes in their health and wellness.

It is the desire and position of the author(s)that you begin to use your intuition about what is and isn't nourishing and healing to your ideal level of wellness instead of allowing science and allopathic medicine to solely dictate your well-being. Each person's health requires a unique and individualized plan. To address your body's specific needs, please consult your healthcare provider.

iii

⟨⟨⟩⟩

Preface

We would like to first congratulate you on getting a copy of Black Woman HEAL Thy Self! Whether it was a personal purchase, a gift, or a required reading, we are thrilled you have a copy in your possession! We are so excited to help you on your journey to a healed life. Much of the information found in this text can be used immediately to help you improve the quality of your life.

I have been working in the healthcare field in multiple capacities for ten years. In all of my years of research, either for myself or for my patients (specifically black women and women of color), there was and still is comparatively, little health and wellness information out there for us and by us. Why does that matter? People are people, right? Yes, however, you have a certain level of trust and confidence in the information when you obtain it from professionals who look like you.

The authors of this book have a combined experience of over 50 years of studying naturopathic medicines and personal successes in their health and wellness. We all experienced a pivotal moment in our personal lives that led us to this journey of holistic healing. Now, we want to share this experience with you.

The Statistics

It is no secret that there are health disparities in the United States.

Health disparities refer to the differences between racial and ethnic groups (Cleveland Clinic, 2022). When it comes to various diseases, black women suffer in high numbers. Women make up approximately 13.6% of the United States population, with 7% of women identifying as black. Black women have a higher prevalence of numerous diseases, including heart disease, stroke, cancer, diabetes, maternal morbidities, obesity, and stress-related illnesses (Chinn et al., 2021). Here are just a few of the statistics for the prevalence of disease among black women:

- Black women are twice as likely as white women to develop high blood pressure during pregnancy (Cleveland Clinic, 2022).

59% of Black adults have hypertension. This is the highest prevalence among all racial and ethnic groups (Cleveland Clinic, 2022).

- The maternal mortality rate for black women is 2.6 times (over 60%) higher than for white women (Hoyert, 2023).
- Lupus is three times more common and more severe in black women than in white women (Lupus Foundation of America, 2013).
- Black women have a 50% higher risk of heart failure than white women (Cleveland Clinic, 2022).
- Black women are 50% more likely to be obese than white women (U.S. Department of Health and Human Services Office of Minority Health, 2022).

Change the Narrative

There have been countless accounts of black women dealing with implicit bias in medicine within the United States. A study conducted in 2016 (Hoffman, et. al.) found that almost half of the first, and second-year medical students believed that there were physical differences between black people and white people. These common beliefs stemmed from the 19th-century experiments that were conducted on black slaves by prominent physicians (Hoffman, et. al., 2016). Some of the beliefs include thinking that black people have less sensitive nervous systems, have a higher pain tolerance, and are more resistant to pain and injury (Cartwright, 2004).

In the 19th century, Dr. James Marion Sims, known as the father of gynecology, conducted surgical experiments on black slaves (Wall, 2006). Dr. Sims would wound the women on surgical tables using physical force and opium. Unfortunately for the women, the drug did not alleviate the pain. However, historians believe that they would then become addicted to the drug, creating additional health issues (Washington, 2019).

Unfortunately, these stories of black women dealing with implicit bias in medicine are not just things of the past. In 2020, Amy Mason-Cooley dealt with a medical crisis that left her in pain that she described as "being sliced open with a rusty saw" (Rao, 2020). After Mason-Cooley spent 24 hours in the hospital, with no relief to her pain, the doctors removed her from all medication despite her continued pain and inability to walk (Rao, 2020).

Mason-Cooley told her doctor, "I don't want you to be in control of my care because you are not listening to me," to which she stated that he not only ignored her but also gave a smirk to her comment (Rao, 2020). Fortunately for Mason-Cooley, additional medical staff placed her back on medication and stabilized her condition (Rao, 2020). 29-year-old Sevon Blake dealt with a similar issue when her doctor told her that her abdominal pain was most likely caused by gas, and dismissed any further concerns of Blake's (Rao, 2020).

Enough is Enough

It is no secret that black women in the United States are facing a significant health crisis. At what point does it all end? That depends on you. You have the power to control your health and wellness; after all, you know your body better than any doctor. We know that there are significant changes that need to take place within the medical system, but until then, you can take a stance for your health and well-being.

This book was created with you in mind. It was created with the idea of being able to provide you with the tools needed to find and create true wellness. The information provided in this book can help you begin the healing process using naturopathic medical practices that allow you to take back control of your health and well-being.

Cheers to your health and well-being!

Blessings,
Jendayi A. Stafford
PhD, INHC, CPhT, Certified Herbalist

I

Introduction

As a child and well into my twenties, I never cared about what I ate. My family never really focused on what we ate as much as the portion sizes of what we ate, the time we ate, and the frequency in which we ate. That was the norm for me and most of the people that I knew growing up in the 90s.

I always had a large appetite. I played a lot of sports, so my eating habits and the amount of food that I consumed at every meal were just assumed to contribute to me being active and needing a lot of calories. I was always told that I had a fast metabolism and that is why I could eat what I wanted to and how much I wanted to. Little did I know that this common misconception of food and eating habits would flip my life upside down by the time I was in my twenties.

I joined the military at 22 years old. Let's just say that the military doesn't always focus on living a healthy lifestyle. For most workdays, I ate fast food. When I say fast food, I mean I was eating a McDonald's cheeseburger in four bites and washing it down with a large fry, two apple pies, and a large sweet tea. While on deployment, I ate zebra cakes like I owned stock in them. I ate my weight in ice cream almost every day and was living off Kraft Easy Mac and Red Baron Deep Dish Singles pepperoni pizzas. I was very active in the military, but I was not nourishing my body. I was constantly stressed out most days and neglecting other areas of my life.

Eventually, my body gave out and succumbed to the toxic environment that I had created. In June of 2013, while on the way to our deployment location, my legs broke out in a hot red rash. It seemed to have come out of nowhere. Accompanied by the painful rash, I was in pain to the point that I could barely walk, and I had a fever that climbed up to 106 degrees Fahrenheit. My body was in a state of full-blown inflammation.

In the following chapters, you are going to learn some of the most pivotal pieces of information that took me and my colleagues more than 20 years to figure out on our journeys of healing. You are going to be able to shave off decades of trial and error and research from your journey of healing and well-being.

As you will soon learn, the most important consultation is the one you have with yourself. Healthcare starts with a personal responsibility. So, congratulations on taking personal responsibility. Now, let's begin!

2

The 7 Realms of Being

The concept of the 7 Realms of Being is something that I developed while working as a marriage and family therapist. With so much of my work focused on the care of the mind and emotions it left little time to explore other potential areas of a patient's life. As a therapist, we are not within our scope of practice to discuss in too much detail anything outside of mental health-related topics. We do discuss potential external causes for the patient's current state of mental health, however, it is just to help us identify if they are the cause of the presenting problem. Outside of that, we make referrals to the appropriate providers.

Early on in my career, I realized that the connection between all the areas in which I am about to discuss played too large of a role in wellness to be ignored. Treating the whole person requires at least a basic understanding of all the parts involved. I began studying in other areas of health and wellness. It was during my studies that I developed the concept of what has now become known as the 7 Realms of Being.

The Clock

We are complex machines! Every part of our being is interconnected with one another. I want you to close your eyes and picture the inside of a clock. All of the gears are independent of one another but are interdependent, meaning they are dependent upon one another to work to their fullest potential. We operate in the same manner. Our emotional, mental, physical, relational, environmental, social, and spiritual parts of us, referred to as the *7 Realms of Being*, are all independent parts of who we are, however, they work interdependently.

Homeostasis is defined as "the tendency toward a relatively stable equilibrium between interdependent elements, especially as maintained by physiological processes" (Oxford University Press, 2019). For us to maintain balance or homeostasis within our lives, we must be operating optimally within our 7 Realms.

What are the 7 Realms?

There are 7 major areas in which we operate. These are known as our 7 Realms or 7 Kingdoms of Being. They include the following:

-Emotional

-Mental

-Physical

-Relational

-Environmental

-Social

-Spiritual

Now, these are in no specific order as far as importance, because again, they are all equally important to our maintenance of homeostasis. While researching each of these areas, I was trying to figure out an easy way for people to remember each of these 7 Realms when the acronym E.M.P.R.E.S.S. came to mind. I thought to myself, how fitting is that!

Empress means "a woman who is a sovereign ruler of great power and rank, especially one ruling an empire." It is in this definition that I found so much power. In the process of trying to heal and create whole-body wellness, I was reminded that I have power and authority over my body, and sickness and disease had no reign. Proverbs 23: 7 says "For as he thinks in his heart, so *is* he". The fact that God put in my spirit the acronym E.M.P.R.E.S.S. gave me so much confirmation that I had the power and that it should do the same for you!

Breaking Down the 7 Realms

Emotional. This refers to your reactions to internal and external stimuli.

Mental. This refers to the cognitive, behavioral, and emotional aspects of being.

Physical. This refers to the whole body, both internal and external.

Relational. This refers to the relationships in which you have with others.

Environmental. This refers to the external conditions or surroundings in which you operate. This can be applied to internal conditions as well. For example, the gut and digestive system have an environment that is separate from the external conditions you experience.

Social. This refers to societal and organizational relationships.

Spiritual. This refers to the human spirit and religious practices.

The Gears

All the above Realms are independent parts of our human experience. They all have their separate functions and needs, yet they rely on one another to be able to function at their greatest capacity. Let's go back to the clock. Externally, when we see a clock, we see a beautiful piece of machinery that is fulfilling its purpose flawlessly. Internally, several gears are working in different capacities for the clock to work. If one of those gears gets stuck or slows down, then it affects the other gears. If the gears are unable to work properly, then the clock begins to slow down, and eventually, the clock will stop. The same is true for you! **Your 7 Realms are the gears, and you are the clock!**

So, how do we keep your gears in alignment? Participate in some activities that will help to create homeostasis.....stability between your interdependent elements.

Emotional/Mental – It is important to make sure that you develop positive coping skills. Coping skills are resources used to help you deal with various types of stress. They can either be positive (deep breathing, journaling, etc.) or negative (co-rumination, drinking, drug use, avoidance, etc.). Coping means investing in your conscious effort, to solve both personal and interpersonal stresses to try to minimize and/or tolerate stress and conflict.

Physical – Be mindful of what you are doing to your body! Eat S.O.U.L. foods (Seasonal, Organic, Unprocessed, Local). Make sure that you are getting up and moving throughout the day. Do a 15-minute HIIT, go for a walk, lift weights, etc. Just get your body moving and your heart pumping.

Relational – Try having weekly family meetings. Incorporate weekly family game nights. Set aside a designated date day/night with your significant other, and a separate date for each child. If you are single, these same suggestions can apply to your close friends.

Environmental – You may not be able to control everything within your environment, but control what you can!

~De-clutter your living/workspace

~Rearrange the furniture in your home/office

~Redecorate a room in your home/office

~Plant a garden with flowers, fruits, vegetables, etc.

Make your environment something that feels good to you!

Social – Create a designated time and day each to check in with your friends. Set up a monthly girls'/guys' night out or brunch. Create a monthly/seasonal/or quarterly movie, television, or book review party.

Spiritual – Do daily meditations. Do daily devotionals. Focus on a scripture of the week. Focus on quieting your mind and body and spending intimate time with God.

As you continue your journey of health and well-being, use the 7 Realms of Being as your foundation. No matter what you choose to implement into your wellness regime, make sure that you are nourishing all your 7 Realms.

3

⸎

Mental Health: What is it Really?

Mental Health

Mental health is an important part of our total well-being that is often overlooked. It includes our emotional, psychological, and social well-being. Mental health directly affects how we think, feel, and respond to both our internal and external factors. Our quality of mental health is determined by how well we take care of our stress levels and our response to those stress levels, as well as our level of emotional, psychological, and social resilience.

When our mental health begins to decline, some of the warning signs can include the following:

- Isolating ourselves from people and activities
- Eating too much or too little
- Sleeping too much or too little
- Losing interest in activities you once enjoyed
- Having invasive thoughts that never seem to stop
- Your mind races late at night when trying to sleep
- You are becoming easily distracted

These are not all of the signs of declining mental health; however, these are some very common signs that may present themselves when it's time to take action to regain your mental wellness.

Mental Health Effects on Your Daily Life

Think about everything that you must do daily. Do you work a full-time job? Do you go to school full-time? Do you have a family to raise? Do you drive anywhere throughout the day? Are you required to leave your home and look like you have your stuff all together? If you answered *yes* to any of these questions, then these are areas of your life that could be affected by the condition of your mental health.

If you are struggling to sleep because of mental health issues, then you may not be able to focus in school or at work. If you are experiencing mental fog, you may be unable to operate a vehicle safely. If you are being overtaken by invasive thoughts, then they may begin to dictate the decisions you make throughout your day.

Mental Health's Effects on Your Physical Health

Your mental health is just as important as your physical health. Too many times, people put their mental wellness on the back burner. Your mental health can have a powerful effect, both positive and negative, on your physical health.

The word psychosomatic means both mind (psyche) and body (soma). A symptom that is considered to be psychosomatic means that the illness of the mind is so strong that it causes the body to suffer as well. These symptoms can include shaking, increased heart rates, nausea, headaches, and tightness in the chest. In some cases, these symptoms can be so strong that they create a physical change in the body.

Pseudocyesis, also known as phantom pregnancy, is caused when a woman believes so strongly that she is pregnant when she is not (Cleveland Clinic, 2022). She may begin to develop physical symptoms of pregnancy such as her uterus increasing in size as though she is growing a baby, and her breast may begin to develop milk. In some of these phantom pregnancy cases, the women have shared that they have even experienced feelings of the "baby kicking.

Although mental health has gotten more recognition since the 2020

COVID-19 pandemic, it has yet to reach the same level of priority for people as their physical health. If you set goals for your physical health every year, then set goals for your mental health as well. There is also a need for people to understand that they need a professional in the mental health field. Just as you would go see your medical provider for flu or COVID symptoms or a suspected sprain or fracture, you should seek a mental health provider for feelings of overwhelm, extreme sadness, or feelings of anxiousness.

Mental Health's Effects on Your Relationships and Social Life

Your mind is very powerful. I have learned over the years that how you feel or think about yourself is how you believe everyone else perceives you. This can negatively or positively affect your personal relationships and social life.

When your mental health is on the decline, it can make you lose confidence in yourself, whether you have a strong sense of self-confidence or not. In my book, Beautiful You Are, I and 16 other women shared how our lack of self-confidence affected our relationships and social lives. For me, judgment was passed on to me by others, I began to believe them, and therefore never created the meaningful relationships and level of social life that I craved as an adolescent. It wasn't until I made the conscious choice to take control of my thoughts and perception of myself that my relationship and social life began to change for the better.

Mental Health's Effect on Your Spiritual Life

So many times, when dealing with mental illness, I have heard stories of people being told by leaders and members of the church to pray over themselves. They have been told that everything can be prayed away if you do it hard enough, long enough, and with enough faith. For most individuals who actively participate in a spiritual practice, there is the belief that there is power in prayer. However, this is not what most people want to hear in the moment of a mental crisis, nor is it beneficial to someone who may already have a fragile psyche.

The state of your mental health can affect how you view your religious beliefs. If you are suffering mentally, then you may begin to view your spiritual practice as no longer being fulfilling.

Common Mental Health Diagnoses

According to the Oxford Dictionary, a diagnosis is defined as the labeled identification of a particular group of symptoms. Most mental health providers have proper education, training, licensing, and credentialing to provide a proper diagnosis. Diagnoses are made through a combination of patient-reported symptoms, diagnostic tests, and the use of the *Diagnostic and Statistical Manual of Mental Disorders* or DSM-V-TR.

Although a diagnosis can fall under a broad title, such as depression, there are specific symptoms that separate these diagnoses into more specific diagnoses or classifications, such as post-partum depression and seasonal affective disorder (SAD). In the next few paragraphs, we will look at some of the most common diagnoses and their classifications.

Depression is a common but very serious mood disorder. Depression can cause severe symptoms that affect how you feel, think, and handle your daily activities, such as sleeping, eating, or working. According to the American Psychiatric Association (2022), Depression is defined as a depressed mood most of the day, nearly every day, as indicated by either subjective report (e.g., feels sad, empty, hopeless) or observations made by others (e.g., appearing tearful).

Nervousness and apprehension are a natural stress response; they are part of our embedded modes of self-protection. However, when you are experiencing proportionate levels of nervousness, apprehension, and fear, this leads to what is commonly known as anxiety. According to the American Psychiatric Association (2022), anxiety disorders are defined as excessive anxiety and worry (apprehensive expectation), occurring more days than not for at least 6 months.

If you feel as though you are experiencing any mental health distress, please reach out to a professional for help. I know that this is easier said than done. There are so many people out there who claim to be an expert in mental health, but who is qualified? The next chapter will

provide a breakdown of the different types of mental health professionals, their level of education, and their scope of practice.

4

Mental Health Professionals

In the field of mental health, there are many different types of mental health professionals. Just about every mental health professional must have a college degree. A few individuals within other professions hold what is known as a mental health first aid certification, but that is not the same as being licensed or educated in the mental health field.

The Bachelor's Degree

At the bachelor's level of education, you will find that these individuals hold a bachelor's degree in either psychology, social work, social sciences, or behavioral sciences. At this level of education, most of these mental health professionals work strictly under the supervision of another mental health provider who is either licensed, holds a higher level of education, or all of the above. An example of this level of professionalism is as follows:

*John Smith, BA (Bachelor of Arts)
*John Smith, BS (Bachelor of Science)
*John Smith, BSW (Bachelor of Social Work)

Again, a bachelor of arts or science degree will be held in something such as psychology, social science, or behavioral science.

The Master's Degree

At the master's level of educational training, you will find that individuals in the mental health field will most likely hold either a master of arts, a master of science, or a master of philosophy. These will most likely be in a field such as psychology, marriage and family therapy, counseling, mental health counseling, clinical counseling, behavioral therapy, behavioral science, or social work. These professionals are licensed, either at the associate level (meaning they can accept some insurances and still require a level of supervision), or they are licensed at the independent practicing level (meaning they can accept most if not all insurances and require no supervision).

Individuals who are licensed at the master's level may work in many different clinical capacities and may work with patients either individually or within a group setting. To become a licensed mental health provider, master's graduates are required to follow the state regulations set by the state in which they desire to be licensed. When I received my Marriage and Family Therapist Associate License in the state of Washington in 2016, I was required to have 2 years (2,000 hours) of post-graduate supervised clinical experience and 36 continuing education units (CEUs) every two years. Mental health professional at the master's level usually has one of the following group of letters behind their name:

*Jane Smith, MA (Master of Arts)
*Jane Smith, MS (Master of Science)
*Jane Smith, MFT (Marriage and Family Therapist)
*Jane Smith, MFTI (Marriage and Family Therapist Intern)
*Jane Smith, LMFTA (Licensed Marriage and Family Therapist Associate)
*Jane Smith, LMFT (Licensed Marriage and Family Therapist)
*Jane Smith, LMHCA (Licensed Mental Health Counselor Associate)
*Jane Smith, LMHC (Licensed Mental Health Counselor)
*Jane Smith, LPCA (Licensed Professional Counselor Associate)

*Jane Smith, LPC (Licensed Professional Counselor)
*Jane Smith, LSW (Licensed Social Worker)
*Jane Smith, LCSW (Licensed Clinical Social Worker)
*Jane Smith, LICSW (Licensed Independent Clinical Social Worker)

It is important to note that the list provided is not comprehensive. There are several behavioral and psychological degrees, and even though the list provided above is extensive, it is not comprehensive. All of the provided professional titles hold a master's degree however they differ slightly in their area of expertise. Typically, an individual who has a master's in psychology has a broad scope and understanding of different theories and therapeutic modalities within the topic. Not every individual who has a master's in psychology is trained in providing clinical counseling unless stated otherwise. For example, I (Dr. Stafford) hold a master's in psychology, but the focus was primarily on marriage and family therapy.

Counseling degrees tend to focus on individual and group counseling. Marriage and family therapy specializes in systemic therapy; they focus on the whole family and other interpersonal relationships. Social workers focus more on getting the individual or family to the right resources, outsourcing things their client may need in a crisis.

Social workers also have clinical training to work with individuals; however, it is not as in-depth as some of the other mental health providers. Typically, the responsibilities of a social worker include case management and hospital patient discharge planning, as well as advocating for their patients and patient's families.

The Doctoral Degree

This is the highest educational level that one can reach. This degree usually requires an additional 4+ years of education, research, and clinical experience post-master's degree. Depending on state licensing requirements, an additional 2+ years of post-doctoral clinical experience may be required. Doctoral students become more knowledgeable in a specific area within the mental health field. Those seeking to work in a clinical setting get additional education and training in the evaluation and treatment of mental health disorders.

Within the mental health profession, these individuals are usually identified by the following lettering behind their name:

*Jane Smith, PhD (Doctor of Philosophy; typically, this will be in some sort of psychology)

*Jane Smith, PsyD (Doctor of Psychology)

*Jane Smith, DMFT (Doctor of Marriage and Family Therapy)

*Jane Smith, DO (Doctor of Osteopathic Medicine, aka Psychiatrist)

*Jane Smith, DSW (Doctor of Social Work)

It is important to note that a D.O. or psychiatrist is the only mental health professional who is initially trained to prescribe medication. The best explanation that I got (which came directly from a psychiatrist I used to work with) is that psychiatrists are trained medical doctors who received an additional year of education focused specifically on mental health. It is important to note that some states do offer post-doctoral training for mental health professionals to acquire the credentialing required to prescribe medication.

Other Mental Health Professionals

Chemical dependency counselor, alcohol dependency counselor. Although these providers are not considered to be your typical mental health provider, they are still trained professionals within the mental health community. A chemical dependency counselor, an alcohol dependency counselor, and a chemical and alcohol dependency counselor are all trained to work with a very specific population. These mental health providers are trained specifically to work with individuals who have been diagnosed with chemical and/or alcohol abuse.

This is a mental health profession that is regulated differently from the others. Depending on the state, these counselors may only require a high school diploma or an associate's degree to get started. These counselors do receive on-the-job training for the work that they do.

Life coach, spiritual coach, and everything in between. Life coaches, spiritual coaches, and any other type of coach are **not** the same as a trained mental health provider! The individual offering services within the coaching field may be trained in mental health first aid or some type of mental health, but typically, coaches are not trained enough to provide mental health counseling. Within the United States, coaches of any kind do not have many, if any, legal regulations as to their scope of practice.

The federal government, state, and different mental health associations have strong regulations and guidelines for professionals in the mental health field. Coaching does not have the same level of guidelines and regulations, which could lead to confidential and ethical issues. The lack of education and training in mental health makes the practice of any kind of mental health services outside of their scope of practice.

Life coaches, spiritual coaches, and any other kind of coach may not be considered mental health professionals, but they are a great and needed profession. Coaches make a great addition to have along with your mental health provider. The addition of coaches can help provide a holistic perspective to your health and wellness.

For more information on any of the professions listed and to find out more about mental health providers, check your state's practicing and licensing requirements. This can be found on your state's Department of Health website.

5

Autoimmune Disease vs. Traditional Disease: Is There Really a Difference?

Let's jump right into why we are here. Discussing disease – specifically autoimmune disease. Learning the clear distinction between autoimmunity and "traditional" diseases. Autoimmune disease is a condition where the immune system attacks the body's cells, tissues, or organs. Autoimmune diseases are specific disorders that result from this misguided immune response, causing harm to various parts of the body. While autoimmunity is the overarching phenomenon, autoimmune diseases represent a diverse range of conditions where the immune system mistakenly targets specific components of the body.

There are over 100 autoimmune diseases, each characterized by unique manifestations and bodily impacts. The increase in autoimmune disease diagnoses with technological advancements is a complex trend. Improved diagnostic tools and awareness may contribute to more accurate identification of these conditions, leading to higher reported numbers.

Additionally, environmental factors and genetic predispositions may play roles in the observed rise. It's a multifaceted issue that extends beyond technological progress.

Here is a list of all known autoimmune diseases:

A

Achalasia

Addison's disease

Adult Still's disease

Agammaglobulinemia

Alopecia areata

Amyloidosis

Ankylosing spondylitis

Anti-GBM/Anti-TBM nephritis

Antiphospholipid syndrome

Autoimmune angioedema

Autoimmune dysautonomia

Autoimmune encephalitis

Autoimmune hepatitis

Autoimmune inner ear disease (AIED)

Autoimmune myocarditis

Autoimmune oophoritis

Autoimmune orchitis

Autoimmune pancreatitis

Autoimmune retinopathy

Autoimmune urticaria

Axonal & neuronal neuropathy (AMAN)

B

Baló disease

Behcet's disease

Benign mucosal pemphigoid (Mucous membrane pemphigoid)

Bullous pemphigoid

C

Castleman disease (CD)

Celiac disease

Chagas disease

Chronic inflammatory demyelinating polyneuropathy (CIDP)

Chronic recurrent multifocal osteomyelitis (CRMO)

Churg-Strauss syndrome (CSS) or Eosinophilic granulomatosis (EGPA)

Cicatricial pemphigoid

Cogan's syndrome

Cold agglutinin disease

Complex regional pain syndrome (formerly known as reflex sympathetic dystrophy)

Congenital heart block

Coxsackie myocarditis

CREST syndrome

Crohn's disease

D

Dermatitis herpetiformis

Dermatomyositis

Devic's disease (neuromyelitis optica)

Discoid lupus

Dressler's syndrome

E

Endometriosis

Eosinophilic esophagitis (EoE)

Eosinophilic fasciitis

Erythema nodosum

Essential mixed cryoglobulinemia

Evans syndrome

F

Fibromyalgia

Fibrosing alveolitis

G

Giant cell arteritis (temporal arteritis)

Giant cell myocarditis

Glomerulonephritis

Goodpasture's syndrome

Granulomatosis with polyangiitis

Graves' disease

Guillain-Barre syndrome

H

Hashimoto's thyroiditis

Hemolytic anemia

Henoch-Schonlein purpura (HSP)

Herpes gestationis or pemphigoid gestationis (PG)

Hidradenitis suppurativa (HS) (Acne inversa)

I

IgA nephropathy

IgG4-related sclerosing disease

Immune thrombocytopenic purpura (ITP)

Inclusion body myositis (IBM)

Interstitial cystitis (IC)

J

Juvenile arthritis

Juvenile diabetes (Type 1 diabetes)

Juvenile myositis (JM)

K

Kawasaki disease

L

Lambert-Eaton syndrome

Lichen planus

Lichen sclerosus

Ligneous conjunctivitis

Linear IgA disease (LAD)

Lupus Lyme disease chronic

M

Meniere's disease

Microscopic polyangiitis (MPA)

Mixed connective tissue disease (MCTD)

Mucha-Habermann disease

Multifocal motor neuropathy (MMN) or MMNCB

Multiple sclerosis
Myasthenia gravis
Myelin oligodendrocyte glycoprotein antibody disorder
Myositis
N
Narcolepsy
Neonatal lupus
Neuromyelitis optica / devic disease
Neutropenia
O
Ocular cicatricial pemphigoid
Optic neuritis
P
Palindromic rheumatism (PR)
  PANDAS (Pediatric autoimmune neuropsychiatric disorders associated with streptococcus infections)
Paraneoplastic cerebellar degeneration (PCD)
Paroxysmal nocturnal hemoglobinuria (PNH)
Pars planitis (peripheral uveitis)
Parsonage-Turner syndrome
Pemphigus
Peripheral neuropathy
Perivenous encephalomyelitis
Pernicious anemia (PA)
  POEMS syndrome
Polyarteritis nodosa
Polyglandular syndromes type I, II, III
Polymyalgia rheumatica
Polymyositis Postmyocardial infarction syndrome
Postpericardiotomy syndrome
Primary biliary cholangitis
Primary sclerosing cholangitis
Progesterone dermatitis
Progressive hemifacial atrophy (PHA)

Parry Romberg syndrome
Psoriasis
Psoriatic arthritis
Pulmonary Alveolar Proteinosis (PAP)
Pure red cell aplasia (PRCA)
Pyoderma gangrenosum
Q
No Results
R
Raynaud's phenomenon
Reactive arthritis
Relapsing polychondritis
Restless legs syndrome (RLS)
Retroperitoneal fibrosis
Rheumatic fever
Rheumatoid arthritis
S
Sarcoidosis
Schmidt syndrome or Autoimmune polyendocrine syndrome type II
Scleritis
Scleroderma
Sjögren's
Stiff person syndrome (SPS)
Susac's syndrome
Sympathetic ophthalmia (SO)
T
Takayasu's arteritis
Temporal arteritis/giant cell arteritis
Thrombocytopenic purpura (TTP)
Thrombotic thrombocytopenic purpura (Ttp)
Thyroid Eye Disease (TED)
Tolosa-Hunt syndrome (THS)
Transverse myelitis
Type 1 diabetes

U
Ulcerative colitis (UC)
Undifferentiated connective tissue disease (UCTD)
Uveitis
V
Vasculitis
Vitiligo
Vogt-Koyanagi-Harada disease
W
Warm autoimmune hemolytic anemia
X
No Results
Y
No Results
Z
No Results

Traditional Disease

The term "traditional disease" typically refers to illnesses or health conditions that are not associated with autoimmune dysfunction. In this context, traditional diseases are those diagnosed based on typical medical criteria and symptoms without involving an autoimmune component where the immune system attacks the body's cells. The diagnosis is concluded from signs, symptoms, medical history, and diagnostic tests without the characteristic autoimmune response seen in autoimmune diseases.

Traditional diseases encompass a wide range of health issues, including infectious diseases, genetic disorders, metabolic conditions, and various other non-autoimmune-related medical concerns.

6

⚜

Healing Is Not A Secret, It's A System

When it comes to health and wellness, people often think that there is a secret to obtaining it. I was one of those people until I realized that it was not a secret as much as it was a system. In this chapter, I am going to share with you exactly what that "secret" system is.

The Mindset Shifts

When it comes to healing, there is a mindset shift that needs to happen. We can have the desire to want to change for the better, but if we don't first have this shift take place, then we will continue to be stuck where we are. What we think becomes what we speak, and what we speak then becomes what we believe and influences our behavior. Several research articles show how our words can influence our actions.

In Psychology Today, Dr. Jennice Vilhauer wrote, "Your thoughts, if you think them over and over, and assign truth to them, become beliefs. Beliefs create a cognitive lens through which you interpret the events of your world, and this lens serves as a selective filter through which you sift the environment for evidence that matches up with what you believe to be true."

A great example of this is a story that was shared in the book The Four Agreements by Don Miguel Ruiz. In the book, Don Miguel Ruiz shares the story of a woman who came home with a headache. Her daughter, who had a very beautiful voice, was dancing around singing. Amid this little girl singing and being joyful, her mother, out of sheer pain being caused by her headache, yelled at her "Please shut up. You have an ugly singing voice." These words spoken over this little girl changed her life forever. She grew up to be very shy and never sang again.

Now that you see just how powerful your thoughts truly are, I implore you to make a mindset shift that will prepare you to be ready to implement the three-part system that will help you get to a state of well-being. This three-part system is the foundation for what it will take for you to get to and maintain a state of well-being. There are a lot of different health and wellness techniques that will fit into these three parts; however, it is important that you know and understand the three parts before making a plan that fits your wellness needs.

Commitment is Key

Whenever we get a hold of new information, we tend to become very excited about it. We will go to great lengths to begin the process of implementing our newfound knowledge into our daily routines. However, oftentimes, people can become stuck in the preparation phase, or they go full speed ahead starting on day one, only to burn out and feel discouraged by their results by day 20.

There have been countless times in which I have started a protocol, and then, for one reason or another, I didn't keep up with it. Depending on what the protocol was and what it was for, within a day or two, I could tell that the good effects that previously went unnoticed from doing the protocol were now being noticed for their lack of presence.

So, what is the reason why I couldn't stick to the protocols? Why, after seeing and feeling the results, would I have ever stopped doing the things that were helping me get to my wellness goals? The answer is simple. I was trying to be consistent when I needed to be committed.

Now, I know you are probably thinking to yourself, "Don't consistency and commitment go hand in hand? Aren't they pretty much the same thing?" These were the same questions that went through my head. I saw this quote from Christine Bissonnette that helped bring clarity between consistency and commitment. "Consistency is nothing more than a set of actions done over and over again. The result of consistency, so often done on autopilot, will always be caged by our expectations, but the result of commitment invites something else into our lives. It invites possibility". I know that sounds so philosophical, but what does it mean?

When I first read this, I thought it sounded great, but I was trying to understand what it meant. After meditating on it for a while, God dropped this one word in my spirit: driving. When you first start driving, you pay attention to everything you do and everything around you. You stay focused on staying between the lines, keeping enough space between you and the car in front of you, and making sure that you use your turn signal at all times. Over time, driving becomes like eating; you do it without much thought. This is because you have been consistent with it. Most of us drive to work, the store, the bank, the post office, school, and just about everywhere we go, which requires us to drive. This same consistent behavior that has become repetitive out of obligation is what can happen when you don't have a passion influencing your actions.

The Three-Part Wellness System

You are the CEO of your health! I know that this may seem like an obvious statement, but it is one that many people don't fully apply. We have all been indoctrinated to go to the doctor whenever we feel sick because the doctor knows about the human body and can help us get better. This is only partially true.

When you go to the doctor's office, you tell them what has been ailing you. The doctor then examines you and may order some tests to rule out potential issues. Once the doctor has finished your physical exam and the tests come back, they can see what is going on in your body and begin building out a treatment plan. This treatment plan usually means being prescribed one or more medications. While medication may not be what you desire as far as treatment is concerned, the fact that doctors can conduct tests to rule out specific illnesses is beneficial to your health.

Look at doctors as auditors of your health. They come in and let you know what's wrong with your body, but it is your responsibility as the CEO to make the changes required to get to your desired state of well-being. As the CEO of your health, you call the shots for the making and implementing a wellness plan that works for you and your needs, not one that works at the convenience of your medical provider.

Understand your body (and the diagnosis). Typically, when you receive a diagnosis from the doctor, you are provided with some information about the diagnosis, how it affects your body, and a brief overview of the medication that you will be prescribed. This is the standard practice of medicine in the United States. While it is nice to have the doctor provide the explanations that they do, it never seems like it is enough information. This can often lead you to do your research via Google, and even that can leave you with more questions than answers.

The reason why it is hard for most people to heal is that they don't have an initial understanding of how their body works. So, when sickness and external factors infiltrate our body, we don't recognize the initial attack. This means you can still be feeding illness without knowing it. I know most of you are probably thinking, "I know my body!" however, there is a difference between knowing your body and understanding how it works.

Think about your car. You get in your car and drive it every day or nearly every day. If your car starts making a funny noise or feels different when you drive it, then you know something is wrong with it. Even though you know something is wrong with your car, you don't exactly know what it is. You don't know exactly what it is because you are not an engineer who has studied the operation of cars nor a mechanic who knows how to fix what stops working properly on a car. The same is true for your body. Most of us have not taken anatomy and physiology courses to understand the intricate workings of the human body.

Although it is not part of traditional education, I would suggest studying the human body and how it operates. This will make understanding how the disease is affecting you much easier, especially when it comes to exploring your treatment options.

To say that there is a real disconnect in most doctors spending the time educating their patients on what a diagnosed illness does to the body is an understatement. As stated earlier, most doctors describe the disease and what it does to the body and then send you home with a plethora of information and prescriptions. It is not common practice within the medical field for doctors to explain how the body is supposed to function and what happens to those functions once a disease is present. This does not apply to all doctors, as the medical field is constantly changing, but in my experience, the education of patients still needs improvement.

Understand your options. Once you have received a diagnosis or pre-diagnosis, do not feel obligated to begin a traditional allopathic treatment immediately. Instead of doing the "traditional" one medicine "cures, treats, or prevents" all approach, find what works for your bio-individual needs.

As you read previously, there is more to you than just your physical and mental. Your 7 Realms should be taken into consideration when developing your treatment protocol. Is what you are going to do or use going to be in alignment with what you believe in spiritually? Is your treatment protocol going to help you continue to meet your needs relationally and socially? I know these may not seem like they should matter, but they do.

For someone taking 3 different medications throughout the day may fit their lifestyle better than juicing celery first thing every morning and eating 4 cups of fruit and 6 cups of vegetables throughout the day. The most important thing for you to understand is that there is no one correct way to treat. In the upcoming chapters, you will learn more about some of the different types of alternative practices that you can use.

7

⚮

It's Your Diagnosis. Learn It. Own It!

The Journey

Embarking on the journey of recognizing and embracing a diagnosis is a huge task. It involves confronting the manifestation of symptoms associated with a specific ailment, which necessitates a deep acceptance. These symptoms have the power to disrupt the carefully envisioned trajectory of one's existence. The life currently inhabited may face profound challenges due to the emergence of these distressing symptoms.

Navigating through the emotions that accompany a diagnosis is undeniably daunting. The instinct to defer the responsibility of diagnosis to your physician is a natural response. However, it is crucial to understand that the weight of understanding any diagnosis information does not rest solely on the shoulders of the medical practitioner. While their role is pivotal, the reality of the diagnosis resonates within the individual's understanding.

Establishing a dynamic rapport with your doctor is undeniably crucial in the journey of diagnosis. However, it is essential to recognize that the narrative of this diagnosis is yours to unravel. This process demands active engagement with the details, a commitment to comprehension, and a deep acknowledgment that the threads of your life story are intimately woven into the fabric of your health.

The intersection of medical information and personal experience requires a delicate balance and a proactive approach. The journey of diagnosis is likely to unravel the intricate threads of your life story. Each detail, each nuance, contributes to the larger narrative of your health. Falling into the victim mindset during this process is a common pitfall. It's easy to succumb to the weight of the situation and begin to unravel emotionally.

Imposter Syndrome

Imposter syndrome, a very real and existent experience during any diagnosis, adds a layer of complexity. Acknowledging that these moments of self-doubt may persist even after the initial stages of diagnosis is crucial. The emotional landscape during a diagnosis can be major. It's a place where fear, uncertainty, and vulnerability intersect. While it might be tempting to visit the unpleasant realm of the victim mindset, it's vital to understand that this is a part of the process. Having been through it, there's a relatable understanding of the emotional toll.

There are moments, even after progress, where the unwarranted visit to the victim mindset occurs. Honesty about this ongoing struggle is essential for individuals facing a diagnosis, as it validates the complexity of the emotional journey anyone diagnosed will face.

The Reality of Imposter Syndrome

Imposter syndrome is a real and persistent companion during any diagnosis. Acknowledging the existence of this phenomenon is crucial. It's not only about the external validation from healthcare professionals but also about self-validation. Understanding that imposter syndrome can linger, and occasionally revisits to that uncomfortable space may happen, is part of the honesty required in navigating a diagnosis. However, it's important to recognize that these feelings don't define the individual's capability to own their health narrative.

Despite the daunting nuances of any diagnosis, there is a resounding encouragement I would like to share: Take Your POWER Back!!! especially concerning health. The intricacies of understanding medical information may seem overwhelming, but this is an opportunity for individuals to actively engage with their health. Empowerment comes not only from comprehending the diagnosis but also from owning the story of your health. It's about steering the narrative towards a path of well-informed decisions and proactive self-care.

8

❧

Benign Ethnic Neutropenia

What you are about to read is based on my life experience with a diagnosed condition called BEN (Benign Ethnic Neutropenia) that affects a specific culture of people that can be congenital or acquired. However, mine is genetic based on culture. You will read about how I live with this diagnosis and the steps I have taken to protect my immune system and keep me healthy and safe. Always consult with your primary care physician or health care providers for all health concerns you have and most of all *BE YOUR OWN ADVOCATE* for your health.

Diagnosis: Benign Ethnic Neutropenia

What is BEN?
When this diagnosis was shared with me by my hematology physician, I researched it, even though he did briefly explain the disease. In this chapter, I am going to teach you what I learned.

Benign ethnic neutropenia is a condition characterized by a lower-than-normal number of neutrophils in the blood. Neutrophils are a type of white blood cell that plays a key role in the immune system's response to infections. In benign ethnic neutropenia, the neutrophil count is typically lower than the normal range but not low enough to cause significant health problems.

This condition is more commonly found in individuals of African, Middle Eastern, and certain Mediterranean descent. It is considered benign because it is not usually associated with an increased risk of infections or other health issues. Benign ethnic neutropenia is thought to be a result of genetic differences that affect the production or life-span of neutrophils in these populations.

While benign ethnic neutropenia does not typically require treatment, individuals with this condition need to be aware of their lower neutrophil count and take precautions to avoid infections. This may include practicing good hygiene, avoiding contact with sick individuals, and promptly seeking medical attention if signs of infection develop. So, now you know what it is, here is my experience.

Somewhere between 2016 – and 2017, I was scheduled for my annual physical to include a complete blood count (CBC). When the results came back, my physician suggested that I see a hematology physician. I questioned WHY, and his response was that his white blood cell count was below normal, which was the first time I had received those results from a blood test. Except this time, there was a concern.

I made the appointment to see the specialist at the hospital cancer center.. which concerned me. For my first appointment at the hematology physician, they extracted twelve tubes of blood for testing, and while I was there, I waited for the results, and the results were unknown.

This went on for several years with me being monitored, and every year, I had blood drawn. On the fifth visit, the physician said he wasn't sure how to tell me what my condition was. I responded with – just say it. I have been coming here year after year, getting blood drawn and not knowing why my white blood cell count is very low or why my blood cells are dying as soon as they leave my body. He said, your condition is because you are of African American descent, and we will continue to monitor your condition, and your appointment will be in 6 months. By this time, 6 months had passed, and I was scheduled to see the hematology physician – the country is shut down with COVID-19, and now I have to wait another 6 months to see the physician.

In the meantime, I am seeing my primary physician on other health concerns. While at one of my appointments, my primary said he is going to resume my appointments with the hematology physician, but it's a different physician. I scheduled the appointment and met the new physician, and he's asking about records from previous years each time I had blood taken. I said he would need to check with my primary, and he said we need to draw more blood from you. Once he said that, I thought to myself – here we go again with more blood taken with each appointment. So, they extracted my blood and processed it for testing, and I waited about 3 months until my next appointment.

On my next appointment with the new Hematology physician, he gives me my official diagnosis and lets me know it's hereditary and there is absolutely nothing I can do. He suggested that I talk to family members. I called one of my sisters,, whom I thought would have the answers I needed; she had no clue and said anyone who would have an answer is gone. (transitioned). From that point on, it was more important than ever to take control of my health and monitor it daily, searching for answers and researching.

In my research, I found a solution that would help increase my blood count to the normal range – or so I thought. On the next appointment with the hematologist, I shared my research, and his response was, don't do that because it can cause another problem for you... In my mind, NO, it's worth a try. I never told the hematology physician or my primary physician that I was in school studying for my doctoral degree in homeopathic medicine at that time or that I live and practice traditional medicine, and that is where my solution is.

As long as I have this blood disorder, my immune system will always, for the life of me, be compromised. So, now I have two things as far as BEN is concerned, below normal white blood count that only happens in a specific culture of people and a compromised immune system, the problem is my neutrophil white blood cell count. To better help you understand the importance of our immune system and the role white blood cells play in the immune system in fighting off pathogens and diseases.

Below, I am sharing the functions of white blood cells with you.

White Blood Cells

White blood cells (WBCs), also known as leukocytes, play a crucial role in the immune system, which is the body's defense against infections and other harmful invaders. The main functions of white blood cells include:

WBC Functions:
Defense Against Pathogens:

White blood cells identify and destroy pathogens such as bacteria, viruses, fungi, and parasites. They can engulf and digest these invaders (a process called phagocytosis) or produce antibodies to neutralize them.

Immune Response Regulation:

White blood cells help regulate the immune response to prevent excessive inflammation or immune reactions. They also play a role in signaling other immune cells to respond to specific threats.

Tissue Repair:

Some white blood cells, such as monocytes and macrophages, are involved in the removal of dead or damaged cells and tissues, promoting tissue repair and healing.

Immune Memory:

Certain types of white blood cells, such as memory B cells and memory T cells, "remember" previous encounters with pathogens. This allows the immune system to mount a faster and more effective response upon subsequent exposures, providing immunity.

Overall, white blood cells are essential for maintaining the body's health and protecting it from infections and diseases. Now that you know the functions of white blood cells, next are the functions of my neutrophils, which are a type of white blood cell.

Neutrophils (WBCs)

Neutrophils are a type of white blood cell that plays a critical role in the immune system's response to infections. Their main functions include:

Phagocytosis:

Neutrophils are highly effective at engulfing and digesting bacteria, fungi, and other pathogens. They use specialized receptors to recognize and bind to these invaders before internalizing them in a process called phagocytosis.

Release of Chemicals:

Neutrophils can release a variety of chemicals, such as enzymes and toxic substances, to help kill pathogens. These substances are contained in granules within the neutrophils and are released when the cell is activated.

Formation of Neutrophil Extracellular Traps (NETs):

 Neutrophils can also release NETs, which are web-like structures made of DNA, histones, and antimicrobial proteins. NETs trap and kill bacteria and other pathogens, helping to contain infections.

Inflammation:

Neutrophils are involved in the inflammatory response, which is the body's initial reaction to infection or injury. They release cytokines and other signaling molecules that help recruit other immune cells to the site of infection.

Neutrophils are often the first responders to infections and play a crucial role in the body's defense against pathogens. (This is Key and very important to the immune system).

All this and to learn there is no cure according to modern medicine. There is nothing I can do to boost my neutrophil count up to the normal range. So, what do I do now, I keep my appointments with my hematology physician who is monitoring my White blood cell count and I have created a personal healthy regimen to protect my immune system especially since we are living with exposure to COVID for a lifetime until the powers that be find a method of eradication of COVID.

My Healthy Lifestyle Regimen:

1) I avoid close contact with people who are sick or have infections to reduce my risk of exposure to pathogens.

2) I eat healthy to provide my body with essential nutrients that support immune function.

3) I have attempted regularly to get enough sleep each night to help my body recover and support immune function. The goal is 7-9 hours of sleep per night. (I fail at this; I may get 4 hours of sleep daily)

4) I engage in regular physical activity, which supports my overall health and immune function. I am a line dancer and I walk about 2.5 hours per day 5 days per week.

5) I keep my primary care physician and specialist appointments to manage my health condition.

6) Take control of my health by educating myself, seeking resources, and creating a traditional healthcare regimen with natural remedies and complementary medicine that is just as effective as allopathic medicine. And since I included this... below are the herbs that I use to make my teas for their immune-supportive properties.

Echinacea Tea:

Echinacea is often thought to stimulate the immune system.

Astragalus Tea:

Astragalus is an herb used in traditional Chinese medicine and is believed to have immune-boosting properties.

Garlic:

Garlic is known for its antimicrobial and immune-enhancing properties. It is often used to support immune function.

Green Tea:

Green tea is rich in antioxidants, particularly catechins, which may have immune-modulating effects. It has been studied for various health benefits, including its potential to support the immune system.

Ginger Tea:

Ginger has anti-inflammatory and antioxidant properties. While it may not directly increase neutrophil counts, it can contribute to my overall immune health.

Elderberry:

Elderberry is rich in antioxidants and is believed to have immune-boosting properties. It is often used to help prevent and treat colds and flu.

Turmeric Tea:

Curcumin, the active compound in turmeric, has anti-inflammatory and antioxidant properties. Turmeric tea is believed to have immune-supportive effects.

Licorice Root Tea:

Licorice root has been used in traditional medicine for its potential immune-modulating properties. Consume this tea in moderation due to potential side effects.

This is me...my life with BEN. If you have Benign Ethnic Neutropenia or know of someone who does... share my story with them and the teas that may be beneficial to them...However, always consult with your primary care physician or healthcare provider for your health concerns.

Thank You for your time and #stayhealthy

Dr. Carolyn

9

Chronic Kidney Disease (CKD)

What you are about to read is based on my life experience with kidney disease. You will read about how I live with chronic kidney disease and the steps I have taken in being an advocate for my health to keep me healthy and hopefully never on dialysis. Always consult with your primary care physician or health care providers for all health concerns you have and most of all BE YOUR OWN ADVOCATE for your health.

What is Chronic Kidney Disease, AKA CKD?

Chronic kidney disease (CKD) is characterized by persistently abnormal kidney blood tests, urine tests, or imaging results lasting for at least 3 months. *Often referred to as a "silent disease,"* CKD typically presents no symptoms until it reaches an advanced stage.

Chronic kidney disease (CKD) is a long-term condition where the kidneys are unable to function properly. The kidneys play a crucial role in filtering waste products and excess fluids from the blood, which are then excreted as urine. In CKD, the kidneys gradually lose their ability to filter blood effectively, leading to a buildup of waste products and fluids in the body.

CKD is often asymptomatic in its early stages and may only be detected through routine blood or urine tests. As the disease progresses, symptoms such as fatigue, swelling in the legs and ankles, foamy or bloody urine, and increased or decreased urination may occur. (*This hasn't happened – at least not yet*).

CKD is classified into five stages based on the level of kidney function, with stage 1 being the mildest and stage 5 being the most severe (also known as end-stage renal disease or ESRD). Treatment for CKD aims to slow the progression of the disease, manage symptoms, and prevent complications. This may include lifestyle changes, medication, and in severe cases, dialysis or kidney transplantation.

Common causes of CKD include diabetes, high blood pressure, glomerulonephritis, and polycystic kidney disease. Early detection and management of underlying conditions can help prevent or delay the progression of CKD. (*None of these causes apply to me*)

Diagnosis: Chronic Kidney Disease

Back in 2020 while at a specialist office, the physicians shared my health report with me and also stated that I wasn't supposed to see the report. I was at this specialist's office for a separate incident that has totally nothing to do with my primary health. After treatment, I took the report, left his office, and went to my car. While in the car, I read the report, and instantly, I got very angry. I questioned myself. Why didn't my primary physician tell me that I had chronic kidney disease?

When he did tell me his back was turned to me as he was reading his report and said, you have only one kidney functioning. I asked how, and I eat healthy and live a holistic lifestyle. His response was, I was probably born with one kidney functioning and just never knew it. I cried, and he asked, why are you crying, and I told him again. I live a healthy life, so what could I have done to have only one kidney functioning?

He said to drink plenty of water, and it will be monitored. Over the years and on appointments, I would ask him, will I end up on a dialysis machine as I get older? He did not have an answer for me, other than it would be monitored.

I researched all I could on kidney disease and researched how not to die of kidney disease. Went back to my medical books and researched the Urinary System and its pathologies. I looked up the Kidney Foundation on Google to read and learn as much as I could about kidney disease. I didn't know that there are five stages of kidney disease, and I listed them below for your information.

Stages of Chronic Kidney Disease (CKD)

Chronic Kidney Disease is classified into five stages based on the estimated glomerular filtration rate (eGFR), which indicates the percentage of normal kidney function. Below is an overview of each stage:

Stage 1 (eGFR 90 or greater): This is the mildest form of CKD, often characterized by abnormal kidney urine tests or imaging.

Stage 2 (eGFR between 60 and 89): Similar to stage 1, this stage is mild and may be attributed to normal aging. Patients may have abnormal kidney blood tests, urine tests, or imaging.

Stage 3a (eGFR between 45 and 59): There is a moderate decrease in kidney function in this stage. Patients often have abnormal kidney blood tests, urine tests, and imaging. Many are referred to a nephrologist for further management.

Stage 3b (eGFR between 30 and 44): This stage indicates a more significant decrease in kidney function compared to stage 3a, with similar symptoms and management strategies.

Stage 4 (eGFR between 15 and 29): This is an advanced stage of CKD, characterized by abnormal kidney function tests and imaging. Patients are educated on advanced kidney disease and dialysis options.

Stage 5 (eGFR less than 15): This is the most advanced stage of CKD, indicating severe kidney dysfunction. Patients discuss their goals for kidney care, including kidney transplant and dialysis options, with their nephrologist.

I have no idea what stage of Kidney disease I have; it was never told to me. I recently learned of the five stages as of today, 2/20/24, and I have been living with kidney disease for about four years. I recently had my annual wellness appointment, which requires a lot of assessment tests, so I will be waiting on all my test results. now that I know about the five stages of kidney disease, I will be asking my primary what stage my kidney disease is. I have previously asked for a copy of my medical records of treatment and know that according to the HIPPA law, you, as a patient, have every right to request your medical records without an explanation. You will have to sign release papers releasing the records and images to yourself... but they have to release them once you sign the Release Papers.

Moving On – So, what do I do living with Chronic Kidney Disease?

1) Drinking plenty of water helps the kidneys flush out toxins and waste products from the body.

2) My nutritional regimen includes fruits, vegetables, whole grains, and lean proteins, which help support my kidney health. I avoid excessive salt, sugar, and processed foods. It took me a while to give up sugar. It was hard, but I did it, and the process was easy to follow. The benefits of following the process led to the near elimination of my desire for sugar.

3) My blood pressure has never been high. It's always low.

4) Maintaining a healthy weight used to be difficult for me because I would eat after 8:00 pm because of my busy schedule. However, I can say that within the last year, I have made it a point not to eat after 8:00 pm. In addition, since I started walking for 2 -3 hours per day, I have lost a lot of weight, but it is within the weight category according to my age, 64 years young.

5) For me, regular exercise is my line dancing and my walking. Regular physical activity can help improve overall health, including kidney function. Aim for at least 30 minutes of moderate exercise most days of the week.

6) My kidney function is monitored on an annual basis because I request the tests to see where I am and how my one kidney is doing. I

am still researching how I can get my other kidney to start functioning again. Even though I was told, it was not possible.

7) There are certain medications I cannot take, such as NSAIDs: Nonsteroidal anti-inflammatory drugs (NSAIDs) can be hard on the kidneys.

For your knowledge: How you can help your kidney health

High blood pressure can damage the kidneys over time. Monitor your blood pressure regularly and follow your healthcare provider's recommendations for management.

High blood sugar levels can damage the kidneys. If you have diabetes, it's important to manage your blood sugar levels through diet, exercise, and medication as prescribed.

Being overweight can increase the risk of kidney disease. Aim to maintain a healthy weight through a balanced diet and regular exercise.

Excessive alcohol consumption can put a strain on the kidneys. Limit alcohol intake to moderate levels.

Avoid Smoking: Smoking can damage blood vessels and reduce blood flow to the kidneys. If you smoke, consider quitting to protect your kidney health.

Monitor Your Kidney Function If you have risk factors for kidney disease, such as diabetes or high blood pressure, talk to your healthcare provider about regular kidney function tests.

A list of Herbal teas for Kidney Health

NOTE: While these herbal teas are generally considered safe for most people, they may interact with certain medications or conditions. It's important to consult with a healthcare provider before using herbal teas, especially if you have kidney disease or are taking medications.

The herbal teas that are **BOLD** type are the teas I make and drink regularly made with honey. The rest listed are herbal teas that are also good for kidney health.

Dandelion Root Tea: Dandelion root is believed to have diuretic properties, which may help increase urine production and promote kidney health. It is also rich in antioxidants.

Nettle Leaf Tea: Nettle leaf is often used to support kidney health due to its diuretic properties and potential ability to reduce inflammation.

Marshmallow Root Tea: Marshmallow root is believed to have a soothing effect on the urinary tract and may help reduce inflammation in the kidneys.

Ginger Tea: Ginger is known for its anti-inflammatory properties and may help reduce inflammation in the kidneys. It is also a warming herb that can promote circulation and is good for digestion.

Cleavers Tea: Cleavers are believed to have diuretic properties and may help support kidney health by increasing urine production and flushing out toxins.

Turmeric Tea: Turmeric is a potent anti-inflammatory herb that may help reduce inflammation in the kidneys and protect against kidney damage. (I also use the turmeric powder)

Corn Silk Tea: Corn silk is believed to have diuretic properties and may help support kidney health by increasing urine flow and promoting the elimination of toxins.

10

Steps to Putting You Back
Together Again

While it is a common practice to diagnose and categorize health conditions, I believe, professionally, that such classifications often overlook the underlying causes of dysfunction within the body. Vitamins and minerals play a crucial role in maintaining optimal bodily functions, and their deficiency can manifest as symptoms that are commonly associated with various diseases. Understanding the importance of these essential nutrients is paramount in addressing the root cause of health issues rather than merely treating symptoms.

Vitamin A, for instance, is essential for vision, immune function, and skin health. Its deficiency can lead to night blindness and other vision-related problems. Similarly, the B-complex vitamins contribute to energy metabolism, nervous system function, and red blood cell formation. Inadequate intake may result in fatigue, neurological issues, and anemia.

Vitamin C is renowned for its antioxidant properties and its role in collagen synthesis. Deficiency can lead to scurvy, characterized by fatigue, joint pain, and weakened immunity.

Vitamin D is vital for bone health and immune function, with its deficiency linked to conditions like rickets and increased susceptibility to infections.

Vitamin E acts as an antioxidant, protecting cells from oxidative stress. Its deficiency can contribute to muscle weakness and neurological problems.

Vitamin K is crucial for blood clotting and bone metabolism; insufficient levels may lead to bleeding disorders and weakened bone density.

Moving beyond vitamins, minerals like calcium are essential for bone and tooth strength, muscle function, and blood clotting. Iron is critical for oxygen transport in the blood, and its deficiency can result in anemia and fatigue. Magnesium plays a role in muscle and nerve function and maintaining heart rhythm.

Understanding the intricate connections between these nutrients and bodily functions is crucial for a holistic approach to health. Instead of merely categorizing symptoms as diseases, addressing the root cause often involves ensuring a balanced intake of essential vitamins and minerals. This perspective encourages a shift from symptom management to proactive health maintenance, fostering overall well-being and preventing the onset of various health conditions.

1. **Breathe**

Taking intentional and deep breaths is not only essential for oxygenating your body but also serves as a powerful tool for stress management. Incorporating mindful breathing techniques into your routine can help reduce anxiety, improve focus, and promote overall mental well-being.

2. **Learn what your body needs**

Understanding your body's unique requirements, whether it's related to nutrition, sleep, or activity, empowers you to make informed lifestyle choices. This knowledge allows for personalized health practices that cater to your specific needs, contributing to long-term well-being.

3. **Listen to your body**

Tuning into your body's signals and responding appropriately is a fundamental aspect of self-care. Recognizing when you need rest, nourishment, or a break helps prevent burnout and fosters a more harmonious relationship between your physical and mental well-being.

4.**Understand there is no one size fits all when it comes to health**

Acknowledging and embracing the uniqueness of individuals in terms of their biology, genetics, and lifestyle is essential. Health is a personalized journey, and what works for one person may not necessarily work for another. Tailoring health practices to your individual needs promotes more effective and sustainable results.

5. **Test your vitamin levels**

Regularly assessing your vitamin levels through blood tests ensures that you are meeting your body's specific nutritional requirements. This proactive approach allows for timely adjustments in your diet or supplementation, preventing potential deficiencies and associated health issues.

6. **Eat Proper Foods For Nourishment**

Choosing nutrient-dense foods that provide essential vitamins, minerals, and other vital nutrients is foundational for maintaining good health. A well-balanced diet supports overall bodily functions, energy levels, and immune system strength.

7. ** Restore Your Cells**

Recognizing the importance of cellular health is key to overall well-being. Practices such as adequate sleep, hydration, and stress management contribute to cellular restoration, promoting optimal functioning of organs and systems within the body.

8. **Regular Exercise**

Regular physical activity is crucial for maintaining cardiovascular health, muscle strength, and flexibility. Exercise is not just about physical fitness; it also positively impacts mental health by releasing endorphins, reducing stress, and improving mood.

9. **Create a Healthcare Team to Treat You as a WHOLE Person**

Establishing a healthcare team that views and treats you as a whole person rather than focusing solely on symptoms is paramount. This holistic approach addresses the interconnectedness of physical, mental, and emotional. These strategies address the WHOLE person, not simply the symptoms. Let's address the root.

For a more customizable way to address your disease, go to www.theautoimmunebully.com

11

How To Take Your
POWER Back

The journey of Taking Your POWER Back in *HEAL*th is not simply about understanding the diagnosis; it's about embracing transformative ownership. It involves recognizing the interplay of personal responsibility and medical expertise. This synergy allows individuals to navigate the complexities with a sense of control and resilience. It's an empowering process that encourages individuals to embrace the details, confront the challenges, and acknowledge their role as the primary author of their health narrative.

While ownership of the *HEAL*th narrative is emphasized, it's crucial to highlight the importance of a partnership with healthcare providers. Establishing a dynamic rapport, as mentioned earlier, is not just crucial but harmonious. The collaboration between individuals and healthcare professionals creates a supportive ecosystem for effective management and understanding of the diagnosis. This collaborative approach enhances the overall quality of healthcare and ensures a holistic understanding of the individual's health context.

The diagnosis journey is complex, multifaceted, and, at times, overwhelming. Recognizing the challenges, both emotional and practical, is integral to developing resilience. The call to Take Your Power Back is not a dismissal of the difficulties but an acknowledgment that within these challenges lies an opportunity for growth, empowerment, and a deeper understanding of self. It's a call to navigate through the complexities with courage and a proactive mindset.

In conclusion, the message to Take Your Power Back resounds as a call to action. Recognizing and embracing a diagnosis is not just a passive acknowledgment; it's an active engagement with one's health and well-being. Ownership of the narrative, understanding the emotional intricacies, and the acknowledgment of personal agency within the context of healthcare are pivotal. The journey is ongoing, with occasional visits to the unwarranted realms of doubt and vulnerability. However, through transformative ownership and collaboration with healthcare providers, health coaches, holistic practitioners, and individuals who can help you navigate the diagnosis journey with resilience, empowerment, and a renewed sense of control over your health.

12

❧

Steps to Managing Your Health

Upon receiving a diagnosis, taking proactive steps in managing your health becomes essential.

1. Preparation

Crafting the most exceptional version of yourself demands meticulous preparation! Without it, achieving greatness becomes an insurmountable challenge. To embark on this journey, take swift action – pick up a pen or unlock your phone's notes. Define your vision of success and map out the steps to reach it. Your plan is the key; in it lies the secret sauce to unlock your success! We are creating the BEST you yet – despite the diagnosis. Ready Set Glow...into the BEST version of you – the HEALED version.

2. Mindset

Mindset is pivotal in navigating life's challenges. Your response to obstacles defines you more than the challenges themselves. Cultivating a resilient mindset is paramount – a strong mentality propels you forward, while a fragile one may impede progress. I urge you to foster mental growth for genuine radiance. The mind holds immense power; seize control before your disease controls YOU. I believe in your triumph; now, it's time for you to also believe in yourself. Let's align your mindset for HEALING! In our fast-paced world, where time slips away quickly, our minds seldom find a moment of repose. Introducing meditation, which may seem daunting at first, yet is remarkably accessible. Embracing this practice unveils the profound benefits of mindfulness. Begin modestly, focusing on a single point or concept, and gradually extend your practice. Remember, there's no wrong way to commence—just commence.

Visualization, oftentimes synonymous with manifestation, is a potent tool for shaping your reality. Craft a vivid mental image of where you aspire to be. This clear vision becomes your daily guide; work persistently towards it. Having harnessed the power of visualization personally, I can attest to its transformative impact. It requires gently stepping aside from self-imposed barriers and envisioning the very best version of yourself.

3. Education & Understanding

Invest time in learning about your diagnosed condition. Understand its nature, symptoms, and potential impacts on your life. Gain this understanding for yourself.

4. Professional Guidance

Establishing a collaborative and open partnership with healthcare professionals is crucial. Prioritize their recommendations, communicate openly about your concerns, and attend regular check-ups for proactive healthcare. Your active participation enhances the effectiveness of the doctor-patient relationship. Your doctors must be willing to take the time to explain any questions you may have. It's a collaborative effort for optimal healthcare outcomes.

5. Lifestyle Modifications

Evaluate and adjust your lifestyle as needed. This may involve dietary changes, exercise routines, stress management, and adequate sleep to support overall well-being. The saying "we are what we eat" holds. Nutrition plays a vital role in our overall health, impacting the physical and mental aspects. Prioritizing a balanced and nutrient-rich diet is essential for promoting well-being and supporting the body's healing processes. Food is medicine! It's what the Creator created. We are what we eat is a very underrated statement. Junk in - disease out. It's just that simple.

6. Exercise

Body movement is another very important part of our healing journey. There is absolutely no healing without movement. Exercise gets the body "flowing". Circulation plays a vital role. When the body is moving, circulation increases. Allowing the blood to flow and carry the nutrients to every cell in your body. Remember, you can be eating all the right things for your body; however, if circulation is blocked, your body isn't getting the proper nourishment. Do yourself a favor and move your body!!

7. Support Network

Build a support system with friends, family, or support groups. Sharing your journey can provide emotional support and valuable insights.

8. Monitoring Symptoms

Keep track of your symptoms and report changes. Regular monitoring can aid in the early detection of potential issues. Pay attention.

9. ?WHY?

Last but most importantly, you have to always remember your WHY. Why do you want to be healthy? What drives you daily? That is your why! You are going to want to highlight this reason. It will naturally become your reason to fight for your HEALth daily. You will think of this very important factor when you are executing all other keys to healing! This journey won't be easy, but it will most definitely be worth it. You have to remain committed and NEVER cheat on your why!!

EMOTIONS

We are rarely taught the physiology of disease. It comes as absolutely no surprise that the emotional portion of disease is foreign to us. It seems as if the paradigm is surreal. However, I experienced it myself: emotions are connected to the human body. We store energy. That stored energy can manifest in your body as a symptom. "We have learned that trauma is not just an event that took place sometime in the past; it is also the imprint left by that experience on mind, brain, and body. This imprint has ongoing consequences for how the human organism manages to survive in the present.

Trauma results in a fundamental reorganization of the way the mind and brain manage perceptions. It changes not only how we think and what we think about, but also our very capacity to think." Ultimately changing the physiology of what our body is made of. The relationship between the mind and the body has been a subject of fascination for centuries. One often overlooked concept in the realm of medicine is the idea that our mental state can influence, if not directly contribute to, the manifestation of physical symptoms. This brings forth a question: can we inflict our own symptoms or at least play a significant role?

Psychosomatic disorders, where mental and emotional factors contribute to physical symptoms, offer a compelling perspective. Stress, anxiety, and unresolved emotional issues can potentially manifest as bodily ailments. The mind-body connection is intricate, and studies suggest that our thoughts and emotions can impact our immune system, hormonal balance, and overall well-being.

Consider the placebo effect, a phenomenon where a patient experiences real physiological changes due to the belief that a treatment is effective, even if it's a sugar pill. This highlights the powerful role of the mind in shaping our physical experiences. While not all symptoms are self-inflicted, understanding this mind-body interplay is crucial in comprehending the complexity of disease.

Moreover, the concept of the "nocebo" effect is equally noteworthy. Negative expectations and beliefs about a treatment or diagnosis can lead to the worsening of symptoms or the emergence of new ones. In this case, the mind becomes an unwitting participant in the progression of illness.

The Emotional Roller Coaster of Disease Diagnosis

Navigating the landscape of disease diagnosis is akin to embarking on an emotional roller coaster. From the initial suspicion to the confirmation or negation of a medical condition, individuals experience a whirlwind of emotions.

The first drop on this roller coaster is often fear and anxiety triggered by symptoms that may be mysterious or alarming. As the diagnostic process unfolds, there's a climb towards hope when considering less severe possibilities. However, this hope is tinged with uncertainty, and the descent can be steep when faced with a challenging diagnosis.

The loop-de-loops represent the various tests and medical procedures, each bringing a mix of anticipation and dread. Waiting for results intensifies the emotional journey, creating a sense of vulnerability and helplessness. Positive news is met with relief, while a negative outcome can lead to grief, anger, and the need for coping mechanisms.

Ultimately, the roller coaster ride may end with a diagnosis that continues into the realm of treatment decisions. The highs and lows persist as individuals decide the impact of their medical condition on their lives and those around them. The emotional roller coaster of diagnosis underscores the need for support, including psychological and emotional well-being, to navigate this challenging time.

13

⚮

Girl, You Got Some Good Hair!

How it All Began: The Early Years

"Natalie, come on let me finish your hair before you go to school for fourth grade picture day." I run downstairs excitedly, knowing I will be the most beautiful girl that day. My mother removes the pink and green sponge rollers. While standing in the living with a huge smile, knowing my hair is going to be so beautiful....Then, I felt a brush or comb go through my hair, and it felt as if my curls needed to be styled. My sweet Heavenly Father, I wanted to pass out right then and there. I did not have a relax at the time and I could feel how my hair went from sleek curls to fro. I said, "NOOOOO!" I moved very quickly from under whatever styling tool she was using to see what happened in real life.

I cried and headed to school. While walking to school I knew the jokes would start but I didn't allow how distraught my feelings to show. It was time to take my school picture and the young black female teachers tried to tame the fro...nope! Nothing worked. So, the next order of business was to self-sabotage my forever picture. To this day relive this moment and laugh at how my mom tried.

A pivotal moment in my life that catapulted my hidden desire to enhance the beauty or handsome features of a person. I started creating hairstyles on my hair from hair magazines or actresses. Every day was a new hairstyle. I had to retire my sisters from putting ponytails and dipping that hard hairbrush in room temperature water. Which was a weekly routine.

Sometime later, I caught a break when my sister's friend was an aspiring stylist who needed clients. I immediately volunteered. She was a good stylist, and it was a new level of hairstyle for me. Her prices were right up my alley $10 or free if she didn't like it. Those were the looks I felt were the best. I was taking mental notes on how she conducted herself while working on an innovative style from scratch. God forbid if the look she was aiming for didn't meet her vision...in the sink, I go with *Pump it Up* holding spray running down my face. She moved on to the next updo with three styles in one. Getting my hair done was a must at a minimum of three times or more a month.

All the skills that I had acquired from my sisters and friends of the family began to ignite a flourishing passion in me, and I was ready to begin creating hairstyles and healthy hair for myself.

Reading for leisure became my way to explore my hair styling techniques. The more I kept diving into my mom's home library I began to become intrigued by all of the natural health books. Books such as *Home Remedies, Vitamins & Minerals,* and *The Complete Guide to Natural Healing* were all my resources for healthy living. I reached for magazines such as *Sophisticate's Black Hair, Hype Hair,* and *Ebony* to name a few. Black hair magazines were my quick guide to creating looks for my family and friends. I was also able to begin exploring how the health of hair is important to creating a phenomenal hairstyle. I did not fully connect with how I could drive my clients, particularly the younger clients, to a healthier lifestyle without any rebuttal

After high school, I was overwhelmed and stressed due to not walking across the stage to receive my diploma. However, I still attended to support my friend because she supported me.

I moved on to Atlanta, Georgia to live to wait on the results of the Georgia State exam in such a frantic state that hindered me from moving forward without a high school diploma. That type of stress caused me as a teen to suffer from several issues such as sleepless nights, facial breakouts, hormones, and hair loss at the crown of my head. While getting ready for work each morning, my hair felt thinner, and the relaxers weren't taking as they should have. I asked my sister to look at my scalp to tell me what she had seen. She was in complete shock. Immediately I began to cry and stress even more due to the lack of awareness of what was taking over my body; STRESS!!!

My next order of business was to go to a salon and cut my hair from uneven strands shoulder length to a short layered bob haircut. This cut gave me a renewed sense of confidence and made me see myself as beautiful which I forgot all about. My results from the exam came in the mail and I passed! All of the weight brought on by the stress of waiting had begun to melt away.

My passion was on hold in the back of my mind due to my new career change in the Navy. Instead of styling other people's hair or nails, I made the focus on myself. Managing my hair and lifestyle became my focus. One of the quotes that I constantly live by is "If my hair, skin, and nails aren't healthy how can I help someone else?"

Healthy Hair is Good Hair!

"Girl you got some good hair!" people would always say, so I walked around believing that. As I got older, I began to learn more about hair health. I attended institutions for trichology and soon realized that I may have what some consider to be good hair, but I had an unhealthy scalp. Overall, it does not matter what the hair looks like, what matters is the condition of the scalp.

Let me better explain this concept using nature. The next time you are driving or walking anywhere, I want you to pay attention to the condition of the trees and flowers. Each of them has its seasons of growing, shedding, and evening blooming. Some will look dry, wilted, strong, full bloom, etc. In seeing the different conditions of some plants in certain areas of your travel as compared to other plants two things could be concluded: 1.) That must be some good soil (scalp) for that tree/flower (hair) to grow that beautiful. 2.) Or the tree/flower must have some strong, healthy roots.

Just like plants, hair goes through different growth phases; four to be exact. These four phases are anagen, growth; catagen, regression; telogen, rest; and exogen, shedding. Let's take a closer look at each of these phases.

The Four Phases of Hair Growth

Anagen. This is the active growth phase in which the hair follicle takes shape and produces hair fiber. The anagen phase is the longest in the hair growth phase. On average, it can last between 3 to 5 years for the hair on your head and shorter for hair growing on other areas of your body, i.e., eyebrows and underarm hair (Roland, 2020).

The *catagen* phase (the transition phase) is the next phase of the hair growth process. It only lasts for approximately 10 days (Roland, 2020). During this phase, the hair separates from the follicle. Although it has separated from the follicle, it remains in place. Approximately 5 percent of the hairs on your head are in the catagen phase at a single given time (Roland, 2020).

The third phase of hair growth is *telogen*, also known as the resting phase. During this phase, the hairs do not grow; however, they do not fall out either. During this phase, new hairs start forming within the follicles released during the previous phase (catagen). This phase lasts for approximately 3 months, and only about 10 to 15 percent of your hair is in this phase at any given time (Roland, 2020).

The *exogen* phase (the shedding phase) is the final phase in the hair growth process. During the exogen phase, hair is shedding away from the scalp, making way for the new hairs that are growing in the follicles (Roland, 2020).

Five Common Conditions of the Hair and Scalp

Most people automatically assume that good hair is based on genetics alone, but that is not the case. Everyone has good hair, but not every one's hair is healthy! Healthy hair starts with a healthy scalp. A healthy scalp will lead to stronger hair and growth productivity. When trying to achieve both a healthy scalp and healthy hair, there are five (5) common conditions to be aware of. Once you learn more about these conditions, you can then begin taking the steps required for a healthier scalp and hair.

Note to reader: Do not self-diagnose; however, consult your trichologist for consultation, evaluation, and recommendations for the prognosis.

Now, let's take a closer look at the scalp.

1. Inflammation of the Follicles.

Follicles on the hair can become inflamed by numerous factors, which include bacterial and fungal infections, physical damage, or chemical damage. Some steps can be taken to help treat the symptoms when this happens. One of the first things you want to do is to avoid any unnecessary physical stimulation. The more you manipulate the irritated area, the more inflammation can occur or worsen.

Another step that you can take to help alleviate inflammation of the hair follicles is to remove or decrease the intake of alcohol. Over-consumption of alcohol can lead to damaged hair and hair loss. The Ethanol that is found in most alcohols acts as a diuretic, pulling water out of the body in the forms of sweat and urination (Davis, 2023). This leads to dehydration of the body, which leads to dehydrated hair. Once the hair becomes dehydrated, it can easily succumb to damage such as split ends, hair breakage, hair loss, and dandruff. Alcohol is also an empty-calorie beverage, meaning there is little to no nutritional value found in it. A person may feel full after consuming an alcoholic beverage; therefore, they have no room to consume a nutritious meal (Davis, 2023).

Lastly, decrease the amounts of greasy foods you consume and replace them with fresh fruits and vegetables. This will help you to increase your vitamin intake, helping to get the proper amounts of nutrients to the hair. Eating fruits and vegetables also helps to hydrate the body; therefore, it hydrates the hair and scalp.

2. Dandruff

Dandruff is a common condition that causes small pieces of dry skin to flake off of the scalp (Schleehauf, 2023). It is a mild form of seborrheic dermatitis. There are several contributing factors to dandruff, such as too much oil (natural or product-based) in the oil glands and hair follicles, dehydration, stress, hormonal changes, and not thoroughly cleansing the hair and scalp.

3. Eczema on the Scalp.

Scalp eczema is a mild dandruff that has a broad spectrum of factors. Metabolic, endocrine, or digestive tract dysfunction, mental stress, intestinal parasitic disease, sweating, and dry skin can all contribute to scalp eczema. External factors that can play a role in eczema on the scalp are chemical agents, cosmetics, spices, dyes, detergents, animal toxins, eggs, fish and shrimp and milk and other heterologous proteins, pollen, dust, bacterial infections, sun exposure, cold exposure, and constant scratching. If you think that you may have eczema on the scalp, please contact your primary care physician for a consult with a dermatologist.

4. Amounts of oil on the scalp.

The stages of oil on the scalp (hair follicle) range from dry to oily. A **dry scalp** is common in the drier seasons due to drier climates, which can cause the scalp to lose a lot of water and increase dandruff. Some suggestions to help treat dry scalp are to get adequate sleep (restores balance and decreases cell injury) and to stay adequately hydrated (our cells are composed of water). Eating an alkaline-rich diet can help balance the pH levels of the skin and scalp.

A too **greasy** scalp can be caused by internal or external grease and fats. These can come from working in a greasy environment (such as a chef or car repair shop). Grease and fats can also come from consuming greasy foods frequently.

When treating an oily scalp, wash your hair more frequently as needed. Use an oil-control refreshing shampoo. As far as diet goes, try to eat light and fresh foods (Mediterranean style diet, whole food diet, etc.). Try to avoid spicy foods. Again, making sure that you are getting enough sleep and drinking plenty of water can help regulate the oil production on the scalp.

Stress and anxiety can also cause excessive secretion of the sebaceous glands in the scalp hair follicles. Life and eating habits can become abnormal when under stress and nutrient intake is not balanced. This may lead to excess oil on the scalp and fragile hair. Never ignore your symptoms. If the symptoms are not treated as soon as possible, the hair follicles will be blocked, dandruff will increase, and hair loss may occur in severe cases.

To reduce your stress and anxiety levels, try to participate in physical activities at least three times a week. Exercise can help to reduce your cortisol (stress hormone) levels. Other ways to reduce stress are to practice deep breathing, practice gratitude journaling, and laughing. Yes, laughing. According to the Mayo Clinic (2023), laughing can increase endorphins, soothe muscle tension, and improve your mood and immune system.

5. Sensitive scalp.

A sensitive scalp shows how the physique is weak. With a weak physique, it is easy to negatively react to physical stimuli such as ultraviolet rays and poor body care products. Most people who think they are sensitive on their scalp are only in a temporarily sensitive state because of the external environment, physiological health, seasonal changes, stress, and other factors.

Suggestions to maintain a scalp healthy hair with a sensitive scalp: you should avoid using very hot water on the scalp, avoid over-styling the hair, and brush your hair too hard. You should also use minimal styling products as they can cause build-up at the root, which can further irritate the scalp.

Your Hair is Your Crown!

If no one has ever told you this, then hear it from me first,

"YOU HAVE GOOD HAIR!" The crown that God gave you is beautiful, and once you learn how to nurture it, you will love it even more! You may not have the healthiest of hair at the moment, but you now have a better understanding of your hair and how you can start to make small changes that will lead to big results. If you are really struggling with your hair health, then I encourage you to seek professional help from a trichologist. You can look up a trichologist in your area using the U.S. Trichology Institute (https://ustrichology.org/find-a-trichologist/).

14

Let's Talk About Food Labels (Not Sex), Baby!

In the world of health and wellness, there is so much information out there on what is and isn't good for us to eat and what level the quality of food should be. In this chapter, we will be exploring what it means for foods to be considered organic and what the food labels mean.

Common Food Labels

Below is a list of the food labels (and their meaning) that are commonly found in the local grocery store (in the United States):

Antibiotic Free. Antibiotic-free means that an animal was not given antibiotics during its lifetime. Other phrases to indicate the same approach include "no antibiotics administered" and "raised without antibiotics".

Cage-Free. Cage-free means that the birds are raised without cages. What this **does not** explain is whether the birds were raised outdoors on pasture or if they were raised indoors in overcrowded conditions. If you are looking to buy eggs, poultry, or meat that was raised outdoors, look for labels that read "pastured" or "pasture-raised".

Free-Range (Free-Roaming). The use of the terms free-range or free-roaming is only defined by the USDA for egg and poultry production. The label can be used as long as the producers allow the birds access to the outdoors so that they can engage in natural behaviors.

GMO-free, non-GMO, no GMOs. Genetically modified organisms (GMOs) are plants or animals that have been genetically engineered with DNA from bacteria, viruses, or other plants and animals. Products can carry these labels if they are produced without being genetically engineered through the use of GMOs.

Grass Fed. This means the animals were fed grass, their natural diet, rather than grains. In addition to being more humane, grass-fed meat is leaner and lower in fat and calories than grain-fed meat. Grass-fed animals are not fed grain, animal by-products, synthetic hormones, or antibiotics to promote growth or prevent disease; they may, however, have been given antibiotics to treat disease.

Healthy. Foods labeled healthy must be low in saturated fat and contain limited amounts of cholesterol and sodium. Certain foods must also contain at least 10% of the following nutrients: vitamins A and C, iron, calcium, protein, and fiber.

Heritage. A heritage label describes a rare and endangered breed of livestock or crops. Heritage breeds are traditional livestock that were raised by farmers in the past before industrial agriculture drastically reduced breed variety. These animals are prized for their rich taste and usually contain a higher fat content than commercial breeds.

Hormone-Free. The USDA has prohibited the use of the term hormone-free, but animals raised without added growth hormones can be labeled "no hormones administered" or "no added hormones".

Natural. No standards currently exist for this label except when used on meat and poultry products. USDA guidelines state that meat and poultry products labeled natural can only undergo minimal processing and cannot contain artificial colors, artificial flavors, preservatives, or other artificial ingredients.

Non-Irradiated. This label means that the food has not been exposed to radiation. Meat and vegetables are sometimes irradiated (exposed to radiation energy) to kill disease-causing bacteria and reduce the incidence of foodborne illness.

Pasture-Raised. This indicates that the animal was raised on a pasture where it was able to eat nutritious grasses and other plants rather than being fattened on grain in a feedlot or barn.

rBGH-Free or rBST-Free. Recombinant bovine growth hormone (rBGH) or recombinant bovine somatotropin (rBST) are genetically engineered growth hormones injected into dairy cows to increase their milk production artificially.

The Great Organic Debate

There is a lot of buzz around the word organic. When something is labeled organic, you would think that it means just that; however, there is more to it than that. Below is a list of the food labels (and their meaning) that are commonly found in the local grocery store (in the United States):

Conventional. Sometimes referred to as industrial agriculture, this describes a system of growing food that uses technology and synthetic chemicals to help increase yields.

Conventional farming may include growing the same crop on the same plot each year (monocropping), genetically modified organisms (GMOs), confined animal feeding operations (CAFOs), and synthetic chemicals that target insects and weeds.

Organic. Food produced through more traditional, sustainable methods that align with the natural rhythms of the land - organic regulations prohibit the use of antibiotics, hormones, GMOs, and synthetic insecticides and herbicides. Organic methods help encourage biodiversity through crop rotation and support mineral-rich soil.

All organic agricultural farms and products must meet the guidelines that are set by a USDA-approved independent agency.

Now that you know the difference between conventional food and organic foods, why should you choose organic food? Here are a few reasons why:

- Organic produce may be significantly higher in antioxidants, particularly in terms of polyphenols(protect the body's tissues against oxidative stress and associated pathologies such as cancers, coronary heart disease, and inflammation), when compared to conventional produce
- Conventionally cultivated produce may have up to 4 times more pesticide residue than organic produce.
- Organic foods/practices help nourish the soil and keep it viable for future harvests.

Organic Labels in the United States

There is more to organic labels than just being declared as "organic." Below is a detailed breakdown of what these *organic* labels mean.

100% Organic
That means the product is completely organic.

Organic
At least 70% of the ingredients in the product are considered organic.

Natural
The product contains no artificial ingredients or added color and was minimally processed.

Certified Naturally Grown
This is a grassroots labeling movement in the U.S. for foods that are produced using organic methods, but the farm isn't certified as organic.

Now, I know that all of this can be very overwhelming, especially when some grocery stores place conventional and organic produce side by side on the shelf. So, how can you tell if what you are buying is truly organic? Let me teach you!

Price Lookup Codes

Grocery stores use price lookup (PLU) codes to label their produce. Foods that are produced organically typically have five-digit PLU codes that begin with the number 9. Conventional produce usually has a four-digit code that begins with a 3 or 4. *It is important to note that not all produce will have this signifying label.*

For example:

Conventional   4011
Four-digit code starting with 3 or 4
Organic   94129
Five-digit code starting with 9

12/15: The Dirty Dozen and Clean Fifteen

The Dirty Dozen. This is the EWG's (Environmental Working Group) list of the most contaminated fruits and vegetables. Purchasing these foods organic is estimated to significantly cut down on pesticide exposure. These are the foods that, when possible, are best purchased organically. The food on this list is:

- Strawberries
- Spinach
- Nectarines
- Apples
- Grapes
- Peaches
- Cherries
- Pears
- Tomatoes
- Celery
- Potatoes
- Sweet bell peppers

The Clean Fifteen. These are the EWG 15 least contaminated fruits and vegetables. These are the foods with the least amount of detected pesticides. These foods can be purchased conventionally if you don't want to buy organic all the time. The foods on this list include:

- Avocados
- Sweet corn
- Pineapples
- Cabbage
- Onions
- Sweet peas (frozen)
- Papayas
- Asparagus
- Mangoes
- Eggplants
- Honeydew melon
- Kiwi
- Cantaloupe
- Cauliflower
- Broccoli

For more information on food labels, feel free to visit the following websites:

US Department of Agriculture. **Food Labels.** https://www.nutrition.gov/topics/shopping-cooking-and-meal-planning/food-labels

National Institute of Aging. **How to Read Food and Beverage Labels.** https://www.nia.nih.gov/health/healthy-eating-nutrition-and-diet/how-read-food-and-beverage-labels

UC Food Safety. **Food Labeling.** https://ucfoodsafety.ucdavis.edu/processing-distribution/regulations-processing-food/food-labeling

15

⟨⧉⟩

The Author's Recipes

In this section, the authors have shared some of their favorite recipes that they use for both themselves and their clients. These recipes are used to help with both specific ailments and overall wellness.

Blue Butterfly Anti-Inflammatory Tea
Ingredients:

- 1 TBSP of dried butterfly pea flowers
- 1 tsp of ground turmeric or a small piece of fresh turmeric root
- 1-2 tsp of raw honey (or to taste)
- 4 cups of boiling water

Instructions:
~Place the dried butterfly pea flowers and ground turmeric into a teapot or heat-proof glass jar
~Boil 4 cups of water in a kettle or pot
~Pour the boiling water over the butterfly pea flowers and turmeric into the teapot or jar.
~Cover the teapot or jar and let the tea steep for 5-10 minutes (let it steep longer for a stronger tea)

~Strain the tea to remove the flowers and any turmeric residue.

~Stir in 1-2 tsp. (or to taste) of raw honey.

Optional: You can add a slice of lemon to each cup for added health benefits such as vitamin C and added antioxidants. It will also change the color of your tea for a very fun visual experience!

Butterfly pea flowers are best known for their anti-inflammatory properties. These flowers are rich in antioxidants such as proantho-cyanidin and anthocyanin, which help with overall health. This tea contains natural antioxidants and anti-inflammatory compounds. Turmeric is well known for its potent antioxidants and anti-inflammatory properties due to curcumin being its active ingredient. Honey not only adds sweetness to the tea, but it also has anti-inflammatory benefits.

Serve warm and enjoy!

Cheers to your health and well-being!

Dr. Jendayi A Stafford

Ginger-Turmeric Tea Recipe

Ingredients:

➤ 1-inch piece of fresh ginger, peeled and sliced

➤ 1 teaspoon ground turmeric or 1 tablespoon grated fresh turmeric

➤ 4 cups water

➤ Honey or lemon (optional, for flavor)

Instructions:

1. In a small saucepan, bring 4 cups of water to a boil. 2. Add the ginger and turmeric to the boiling water.

2. Reduce the heat and simmer for about 10-15 minutes. 4. Remove the saucepan from the heat and let the tea steep for an additional 5 minutes.

3. Strain the tea into a cup using a fine mesh strainer or cheesecloth.

4. Add honey or lemon to taste, if desired.

Enjoy your ginger-turmeric tea!
#stayhealthy
Dr. Carolyn Hubert-Black

Healing Herbal Limeade
1.) 16 oz spring water
2.) 1 TBSP of Hibiscus Herb (put in a tea bag or strain after the water turns dark pink/purple/red)
3.) 5 Key limes
4.) 2 TBSP of Agave

Stir all of the ingredients together and enjoy!

This is a very healing drink. It is important to note that no substitutions should be made. Substituting any of the ingredients will alter the healing benefits of the limeade.

Hibiscus helps with health issues such as poor circulation, high blood pressure, toxins in the blood, flu, cough, sore throat, and respiratory infection. It also helps in restoring and maintaining overall health and is very high in iron.

Immune-Boosting Herbal Tea Recipe
Ingredients:
1 teaspoon echinacea root
1 teaspoon astragalus root
1 teaspoon licorice root
1-inch piece of fresh ginger, sliced
4 cups water Honey (optional, for sweetness)
Instructions:

1. In a small saucepan, combine the echinacea root, astragalus root, licorice root, and ginger slices with 4 cups of water.
2. Bring the water to a boil, then reduce heat and simmer for 10-15 minutes.

3. Remove the saucepan from the heat and let the tea steep for an additional 5-10 minutes.
4. Strain the tea into a cup using a fine mesh strainer or cheesecloth to remove the herbs and ginger.
5. Add honey to taste if desired. Enjoy your immune-boosting herbal tea!

Note: Pregnant women and individuals with high blood pressure, heart conditions, or kidney disease should consult with a healthcare provider before using licorice root.

Dr. Carolyn Hubert-Black

16

Final Thoughts

Congratulations! You have reached the end of this book. It is our sincere hope that you have finished this book feeling more educated and empowered concerning your healthcare. As you continue to create what your healthcare looks like for you, keep this book close by as a resource. Refer to each chapter as needed.

Moving forward we are very excited to announce that Black Woman HEAL Thy Self is just the beginning! We are currently working on other books that will be a part of the *Black Woman HEAL Thy Self* book series. Our next book, a healing recipe book, will be launching in the summer of 2024, so be on the lookout for that. Again, it is our sincerest hope that this book has been an empirical and much enjoyed part of your health and wellbeing journey.

Cheers to your health and well-being!

Sincerely,
Dr. Jendayi A Stafford, Dr. Carolyn Hubert-Black, Natalie Martin, and Anita Monique ~ The Autoimmune Bully

Jendayi A. Stafford, Ph.D.

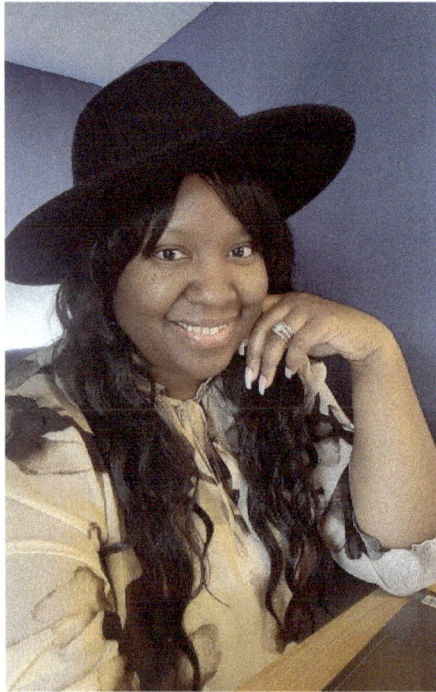

Contributing Author of:
~Preface
~Introduction
~The 7 Realms of Being
~Mental Health: What is it Really?

~Mental Health Professionals
~Healing is Not a Secret; It's a System
~Let's Talk About Food Labels (Not Sex), Baby!
~Author's Recipes
~Final Thoughts

Biography of Jendayi A. Stafford, Ph.D.

Dr. Jendayi A. Stafford, a medically retired Navy veteran, is a developmental psychologist and integrative nutrition health coach dedicated to educating and advocating for holistic healing and transforming the lives of those suffering from chronic diseases.

Dr. Stafford got her start in the health and wellness field out of a personal need. Diagnosed with an autoimmune disease in 2014, she tried traditional medication for over two years. When she became pregnant in 2016, Dr. Stafford began searching for natural alternatives to medication that could be used during her pregnancy. This led to not only a personal lifestyle change but also a change within her career. She had found her purpose!

Dr. Stafford holds a Bachelor's degree in Social Science with an emphasis in Psychology, Sociology, and Criminal Justice, 3 Masters degrees in Psychology, Developmental Psychology, and Organizational Leadership, as well as a Ph.D. in Developmental Psychology. She also holds certifications as a pharmacy technician and integrative nutrition health coach.

Dr. Stafford is one of the dedicated members of Dr. Heather Hamilton's BreakThrough! team. She serves as a member of the Congressional Lead for the fourth district of Virginia with the Americans for Homeopathy Choice Homeopathy Action Team. She also serves with the National Homeopathic Product Certification Board on both the Global and Outreach Committees.

Dr. Stafford's unwavering dedication, expertise, and compassionate nature make her a revered figure in the fields of psychology and holistic healing. Through her profound insights, she inspires and empowers individuals to achieve health, happiness, and overall well-being.

Dr. Carolyn Hubert-Black

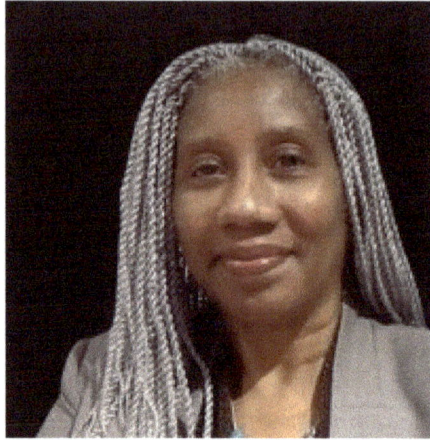

Contributing Author of:
~Benign Ethnic Neutropenia (BEN)
~Chronic Kidney Disease (CKD)
~Author's Recipes
~Final Thoughts

Biography of Dr. Carolyn Hubert-Black

Carolyn Hubert-Black is a dedicated and experienced healthcare provider, traditional medicine practitioner, and educator with over three decades of experience in the healthcare industry. Since 1983, Carolyn has successfully managed two private practices, offering services for both medical conditions and cosmetic procedures. Her expertise extends to teaching in the healthcare field, where she has developed course curricula and state programs for vocational trade schools.

As a practicing traditional medicine practitioner with a focus on homeopathic medicine, Carolyn is dedicated to providing holistic healthcare solutions. She is currently a doctoral candidate in homeopathic medicine, furthering her knowledge and expertise in the field. Additionally, Carolyn is a nationally approved continuing education provider for licensed massage therapists, demonstrating her commitment to ongoing education and professional development in the healthcare sector.

Carolyn's passion lies in educating and empowering individuals to take control of their health and well-being through natural and holistic approaches. Her wealth of experience and dedication to her field make her a valuable asset in the healthcare and education sectors.

Natalie Martin, Trichologist

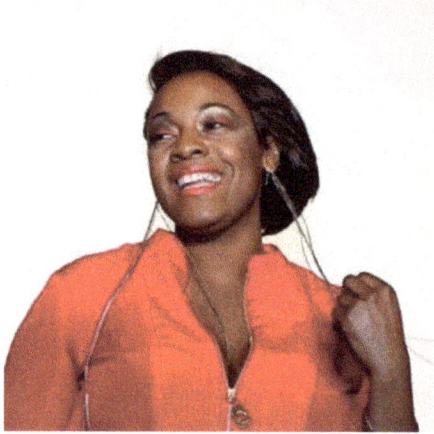

Contributing Author of:
~Girl, You Got Some Good Hair!
~Final Thoughts

Biography of Natalie Martin

Natalie Martin was born and raised in Savannah, GA. It was there that she developed her passion for hair. She is currently serving her 19th year on active duty in the United States Navy and is a licensed trichologist. She is a graduate of the Paul Mitchell Hair & Beauty School of Jacksonville and of the National Trichology Training Institute (NTTI). She also earned her certification in RESTORE!, a comprehensive wellness program. These certifications gave Natalie the tools to share her inspiring journey with the world and to continue to grow.

Natalie is passionate about learning more about holistic health and wellness and immersing herself in the current research in those areas.

Natalie is dedicated to her craft as a trichologist and continues to learn and train with the resources provided by the U.S. Trichology Institute (USTI). She has a passion for serving her country and learning all she can to help her clients, not only with the health of their hair but with their overall well-being.

"If you want your hair to grow, let's start at the scalp." Natalie desires to "Go to the grave empty" because the wealth of knowledge she has obtained over her lifetime would have been shared with those willing to have it.

Anita Monique, The Autoimmune Bully

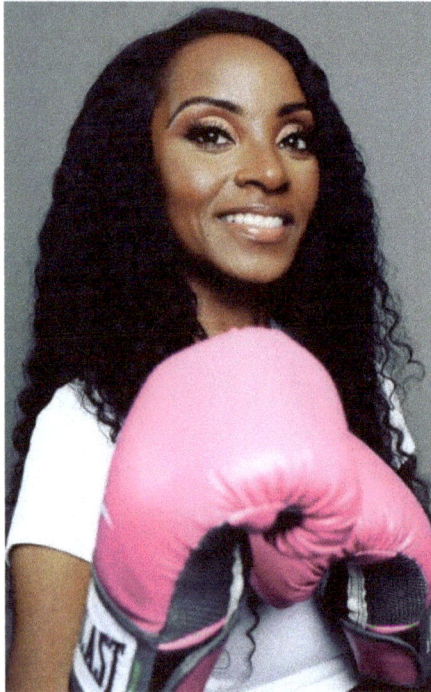

Contributing Author of:
~Autoimmune Disease vs. Traditional Disease:
Is There a Difference?
~It's Your Diagnosis. Learn It. Own It.
~Steps to Put You Back Together Again
~Steps to Manage Your Health
~Author's Recipes
~Final Thoughts

Biography of Anita Monique

I am Coach Anita Monique, a name synonymous with resilience and empowerment. My journey through life is a testament to the indomitable spirit of the human will, a story that inspires and underscores the profound impact one person can have on the lives of many.

In my early life, I had a successful career as an optician. My passion for helping others see the world more clearly was evident in the quality of my work and the joy I brought to my patients. Life was unfolding beautifully until a fateful diagnosis that would forever alter the course of my story—Multiple Sclerosis.

Multiple Sclerosis, a challenging and unpredictable autoimmune disease, took a toll on my mobility. The very foundation upon which I built my life seemed to crumble. But what defines a person is not the adversity they face, but how they respond to it. I chose to respond with unwavering determination. I chose to regain control and Take My POWER Back!!!

Fueled by a relentless pursuit of knowledge and a deep desire to regain control of my life, I immersed myself in the world of regenerative health. I became a dedicated student, learning the intricacies of the human body and the profound impact of holistic healing practices. My passion for understanding the body's innate capacity to heal itself led me to become a Certified Dr Terry Wahls Healthcare Practitioner, coupled with being an IIN Health Coach. I gained valuable insights into the power of nutrition and lifestyle in managing autoimmune conditions.

But my journey didn't stop there. I continued to deepen my expertise, becoming an autoimmune herbalist. My knowledge of herbs and natural remedies allowed me to offer holistic solutions to those facing autoimmune challenges, just as I had.

However, perhaps the most effective and remarkable aspect of my story is my role as "The Autoimmune Bully." This title may seem unexpected, but it portrays my mission: to confront and conquer autoimmune conditions head-on. I emerged as an advocate and became a voice for those who often felt overwhelmed by their diagnosis. I became a beacon of hope, teaching others that they could regain control of their health by confronting and conquering autoimmune symptoms head-on. Urging many to address the root of the disease and not simply the symptoms.

Today I am proudly an advocate and a voice for those who often feel overwhelmed by their diagnosis. I became a beacon of hope, teaching others that they, too, can take control of their health, just as I had.

My journey is a testament to the human spirit's incredible power and regenerative health's transformative potential. I went from a successful optician to a beacon of hope, empowering countless individuals to take charge of their autoimmune conditions and reclaim their lives.

I wish for my story to remind everyone that even in the face of adversity, you can rebuild, reinvent, and inspire others along the way. Living life freely despite my Multiple Sclerosis diagnosis and my personal decision of NOT selecting to take a disease-modifying therapy. It is my dream to create a legacy of strength, resilience, and a profound commitment to regenerative well-being.

References

American Psychiatric Association. (2022). Depressive disorders. In *Diagnostic and Statistical Manual of Mental Disorders* (5th ed., text rev.).

Chinn, J. J., Martin, I. K., Redmond, N. (2021). Healthy equity among black women in the United States. *Journal of Women's Health*. Retrieved from https://www.ncbi.nlm.nih.gov/pmc/articles/PMC8020496/.

Clevland Clinic. (2022). How race and ethnicity impact heart disease. Retrieved from https://my.clevelandclinic.org/health/articles/23051-ethnicity-and-heart-disease.

Clevland Clinic. (2022). Pseudocyesis. Retrieved from https://my.clevelandclinic.org/health/diseases/24255-pseudocyesis

Davis, K. (2023). Is alcohol bad for your hair? Retrieved from https://www.medicalnewstoday.com/articles/is-alcohol-bad-for-your-hair.

Ebong, I, and Breathett, K. (2020). The cardiovascular disease epidemic in African American women: Recognizing and tackling a persistent problem. Retrieved from https://www.ncbi.nlm.nih.gov/pmc/articles/PMC7371547/

Gupta, A. (2023). Does autoimmune disease affect your libido? What you should know. Retrieved from https://www.welltheory.com/resources/autoimmunity-and-libido

Hoffman, K. M., Trawalter, S., Axt, J. R., Oliver, M. N. (2016). Racial bias in pain assessment and treatment recommendations, and false beliefs about biological differences between blacks and whites. *Proceedings of National Academy of Sciences of the United States of America.* Retrieved from https://www.ncbi.nlm.nih.gov/pmc/articles/PMC4843483/#r20

Hoyert, D. (2023). Maternal mortality rates in the United States. Retrieved from https://www.cdc.gov/nchs/data/hestat/maternal-mortality/2021/maternal-mortality-rates-2021.htm#:~:text=In%202021%2C%20the%20maternal%20mortality,(Figure%201%20and%20Table).

Mayo Clinic. (2023). Stress relief from laughter? It's no joke. Retrieved from https://www.mayoclinic.org/healthy-lifestyle/stress-management/in-depth/stress-relief/art-20044456.
Oxford University Press. (2019). Homeostasis. In *Oxford English dictionary.*

Rao, V. (2020). You are not listening to me: Black women on pain and implicit bias in medicine. Today. Retrieved from https://www.today.com/health/implicit-bias-medicine-how-it-hurts-black-women-t187866

Roland, J. (2020). What are the four stages of hair growth? *Healthline.* Retrieved from https://www.healthline.com/health/stages-of-hair-growth

Schleehauf, B., (2023). *American Academy of Dermatology Association.* How to Treat Dandruff. Retrieved from https://www.aad.org/public/

everyday-care/hair-scalp-care/scalp/treat-
dandruff#:~:text=Dandruff%20is%20a%20com-
mon%20scalp,also%20make%20your%20scalp%20itch.

U.S. Department of Health and Human Services Office of Minority
Health. (2022). Obesity and African Americans. Retrieved from
https://minorityhealth.hhs.gov/obesity-and-african-americans

Wall, L. L. (2006). The medical ethics of Dr. J Marion Sims: A fresh
look at the historical record. Journal of Medical Ethics. Retrieved from
https://www.ncbi.nlm.nih.gov/pmc/articles/PMC2563360/

Washington, H. A. (2019). A medical hell recounted by its victims.
Nature Journal. Retrieved from https://www.nature.com/articles/
d41586-019-00340-5#:~:text=In%20the%201840s%2C%20the%20Ala-
bama,they%20became%20addicted%20to%20it.

Wilson, N. (2022). Researchers take a multifaceted approach to
understanding autoimmune disease disparities. Retrieved from
https://medicine.musc.edu/departments/dom/news-and-awards/2022/
may-2022/understanding-autoimmune-disease-
disparities#:~:text=The%20disproportion-
ate%20rates%20at%20which,as%20African%20American%20or%20His-
panic.

www.ingramcontent.com/pod-product-compliance
Lightning Source LLC
Chambersburg PA
CBHW051248020426
42333CB00025B/3111